Praise for
Your Body Lives Your Story

"Ellen Meredith has written a beautiful book that puts into your hands the tools to make conversation with your body and listen to the brilliance coming from inside you. Every part of you is alive with story and emotions, and this internal dialogue with your organs, body parts, and dimensions of self will guide you to your answers and healing. Everywhere I turn it draws me in. This is a book that can change your life."

—DONNA EDEN, author of *Energy Medicine*

"I'm always excited to read a new book by Ellen Meredith, but beyond excitement about this book. It falls under the category: Absolutely Necessary. *Your Body Lives Your Story* explores the intensity of what is going on in our fractured world and how it affects you personally. There's never been a better time to understand and deal with the competing narratives for your attention. How to not get overwhelmed. How to know what to trust. How do you even know who you are anymore? With clear and compelling writing and easy to practice exercises, you'll be able to find internal ease and clarity, which will make every aspect of your life better. Ellen's book is the gift you need right now."

—LAUREN K. WALKER, creator and bestselling author
of *Energy Medicine Yoga*

"Another transformative guide by Ellen Meredith! Inside you will find powerful tools to help navigate the chaos of modern life through the lens of subtle energies. With the introduction of the Storymaker energy mechanism, it provides an insightful journey of self-discovery and healing that speaks to both beginners and seasoned practitioners. A must-read for anyone seeking clarity, personal evolution, and a deeper connection to their own energy."

—SHERIANNA BOYLE, author of *Just Ask Spirit: Free Your Emotions to Energize Intuition & Discover Purpose*

"Ellen Meredith's *Your Body Lives Your Story* is a profound eye-opening and mind-bending guide to self-healing your body, mind, and spirit by weaving through the stories of your past, present, and future. Dive into these incredible lifesaving practices to unlock stuck places, repattern, heal, and evolve yourself. Become all that you can truly be in this lifetime. A fantastic journey awaits!"

—KAREN R. ONOFRIO, MD, certified Eden Method practitioner

"These days, many of us are dealing with bodily issues that mainstream medicine cannot diagnose or treat. In this book, Ellen Meredith shares her deep expertise so we can take responsibility for our own healing and bring it to the next level. The Universe delivers what we need when we ask for it, and this book 'miraculously' landed in my lap at just the right time. If you're reading these words, I'll bet there's a miracle in here for you, too."

—LISA BONNICE, author and host at The Shift Network

"Stories are the essence of who we are. They hold the memories of our journey through this school of life. Whether joyful or challenging, these memoirs become imprinted within our bodies and energy systems. Like scar tissue, they often keep us stuck and prevent us from living the extraordinary lives we so deserve. In Ellen's book, she presents a brilliant and transformative method for connecting with our inner Storymaker. This guiding force invites us to take ownership of our healing and personal growth. By following the wisdom of the Storymaker, we unlock the power to heal, realign, and step into our fullest potential, radiating the light of who we truly are."

—TITANYA MONIQUE DAHLIN, Life Color Intuitive/
Eden Energy Medicine teacher

"This is a book that will get you nodding in agreement—it did me. Why? Because it is truly relevant to the world we find ourselves in today. Ellen inspires with a magical and creative combination of her own storytelling, inspiring insights, all supported by practical 'exercises' to help you discover infinite possibilities in creating a new way of living and being."

—MADISON KING, energy educator and author of *Everyday Energy*

"In *Your Body Lives Your Story,* Ellen Meredith makes a compelling case: your body isn't just a biological machine—it's a storyteller. Symptoms, emotions, and synchronicities all carry messages, waiting to be decoded. Blending science, spirituality, and case studies, she teaches readers to translate these signals into wisdom. If you've ever suspected your body knows more than your mind does, this book is your roadmap to understanding its secret language."

—DAWSON CHURCH, best-selling author of *Spiritual Intelligence*

"Your Body Lives Your Story is a brilliant dive into the mind-body-energy connection, revealing how the stories we create from life's experiences shape us on every level. This essential work empowers readers to recognize this process so that they can find true liberation, alignment and healing. Ellen Meredith has given us another set of keys to the castle of our consciousness—and somehow made it all fun along the way!"

—LISA CAMPION, author of *The Art of Psychic Reiki* and *Energy Healing for Empaths*

"There is so much rich, deep information and wisdom to be mined in *Your Body Lives Your Story.* Ellen Meredith has struck energy medicine gold once again. As an Energy Medicine practitioner, I use Ellen's techniques with almost every client—and they work. Inspirational, educational, empowering and easy to implement, this book will change your life forever. What a gift to the world!"

—DIANNE FAURE, author of *Cancer and Energy Medicine*

"This is a wonderful book. I was hooked from the start. Captivatingly written, it roots important considerations in practical, everyday experiences that we can all relate to. It oozes love, joy, hope, calmness, possibility, and healing. Examples, story and guidance are enriched with a multitude of very do-able exercises that can quickly shift you into insight and inner wisdom about you and your life. Inspiring—and indispensable in these times."

—ALISON PALMER, PhD, founder of the Crones Summits

"Part of being human is our gift of language; we all tell stories about what we have lived, imagined, and believe. What we may not realize is that we carry all of those stories in our bodies, for better or for worse. Ellen Meredith, a master storyteller herself, shows the way to creatively dialogue with our bodies, offering empowering tools and exercises to shift the narrative towards greater joy and health. Enjoy!"

—BARBARA TOWNER, MD, EEMAP

"Ellen's ability to clearly transmit transformational self-healing energy practices is extraordinary! I have been teaching and practicing material from her workshops and first two books for years and have seen their power first-hand. I can't wait to share these new techniques with my students and incorporate them in treating clients. Thank you Ellen, for these gifts and for sharing the process of how you received them. It is truly inspiring!"

—DEVI STERN, Energy Medicine teacher, author of *Energy Healing with the Kabbalah*

Your Body Lives Your Story

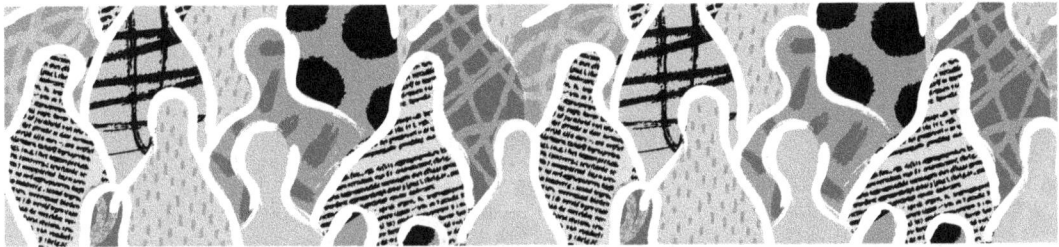

Energy Medicine to Heal Your *Storymaker*

Ellen Meredith

HORSE Mountain PRESS
SAN RAFAEL, CA

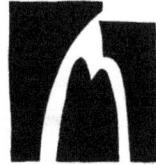

Published by

HORSE
mountain
PRESS

SAN RAFAEL, CA
www.listening-in.com

Disclaimer: All identifying information and details in client responses and case examples have been changed to render persons unidentifiable to maintain confidentiality.

This book is not a replacement for therapy nor consultation with a health professional. Please seek health care from a licensed professional for further assistance as needed.

ISBN-13: 978-0-9636073-0-0 (print)
          978-0-9636073-1-7(epub)

BOOKS AND AUDIO BY ELLEN MEREDITH

Listening In:
Dialogues with the Wiser Self

In Search of Radiance:
Learning to Stand with Your Wiser Self (audio)

The Language Your Body Speaks:
Self-Healing with Energy Medicine

Your Body Will Show You the Way:
Energy Medicine for Personal and Global Change

BOOKS PUBLISHED AS ELLEN M. ILFELD

Learning Comes to Life:
An Active Learning Program for Teens

Good Beginnings:
Parenting in the Early Years
coauthored with J.L. Evans

Early Childhood Counts:
A Programming Guide on Early Childhood Care for Development
coauthored with J.L. Evans and R.G. Myers

To my students, clients, and readers who want to find the flame within to light their way—and who are choosing to co-create a world where all of us can thrive.

May we each find our own inner guidance, World Wise Web, creativity, and moment-by-moment ways to contribute to the well-being of our planet and cultures.

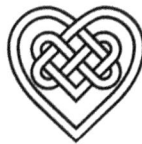

Contents

A World That Makes Sense and Has Meaning

Last week I flunked a *National Geographic* quiz. Under a caption of "Guess which picture is real," it showed two views of a Siberian tiger: an actual photo and one generated with artificial intelligence (AI). The image on the left was head-on, as if posing for the camera. The right one showed a slight side view, the tiger's face turned coyly toward the camera as if just noticing it. Both were in stunning, vivid detail and color.

I was sitting in my favorite recliner, the one where I can see to the right of me the charming rose garden we inherited from the former owners of the house and, ahead of me, what I think of as my magic hill, which turns green in winter and reminds me of Ireland, then turns golden brown in summer, looking more like an African veldt. It's still golden brown here in Northern California as we head into winter.

I came across this quiz while noodling on my phone. My logical mind went back and forth, coming up with good arguments for which image was the real one. Then I thought, somewhat smugly I confess, *I'm psychic—I'll tune in with my Spidey senses to get to the truth.* I chose the coy side view. It felt slightly more believable than the head-on shot because it was less perfect. And I was wrong.

Normally, I am not competitive about little pop quizzes. But I spent several minutes searching for clues that would tell me why I got it wrong. What was *more real* about the real photo? I just couldn't tell. Then I fell down a rabbit hole.

"What does this mean for civilization and the future of our world?" I asked myself. "How will this *not* be used to manipulate people even more completely than we have already been manipulated?" My breathing grew shallower, and all my energy was up in my head. "Is there anyone on duty somewhere who can make sure our world isn't going to be run and conditioned by the sensibilities of Silicon Valley tech bros?" Panic was setting in. I didn't see the gorgeous African veldt or sweet rose garden. I started to blur, and any felt sense I had of a world I want to live in, a world that makes sense and has meaning, began to dissolve.

Then my cat jumped on my lap and stretched up to rub her face on mine. She made muffins on my legs, turned in a circle a few times, and settled in. She knew what was real—a convenient lap. It snapped me out of my fug and made me laugh. Of course, I knew what was real: this small tiger-striped being, sitting in my lap.

I realized it was a trick question: Neither photo was real. Both were probably manipulated, and though both *looked* like tigers, they were equally representations of something not actually in my realm of experience. They were stand-ins for a creature I'd just as soon *not* have in my lap or see for real outside my window.

As we head rapidly into the heart of the 2020s, I'm feeling like an old lady for the first time, complaining about how quickly everything is changing, bemoaning the loss of the world I was used to, which my mom bemoaned as the loss of her world, and so on backward. And I'm in the same boat as many of my friends: struggling with news addiction, having to take a hard look at my relationship with my phone, and the hours I spend reading snippets of opinion and questionable news and the entertainment equivalent of junk food—cute videos on YouTube. (Not that junk food doesn't have its place!)

I wish the answer would be to just detach from my phone. Don't look at it, unsubscribe, stop following all the events around the world that are so horrifying and compelling, like a sore tooth I keep touching to see if it still hurts. It does.

I make excuses: I *have* to check my phone because most of my work is virtual right now. What if someone wants to communicate with me? But the fact is, I've become addicted because of the sheer *volume* and instant gratification of information available to me. I am curious, I keep scrolling, I get hooked in by headlines or teasers, or worse, I get drawn into a pervasive fear narrative that has gotten under my skin: that authoritarianism will take over my democracy if I don't stay vigilant every moment. And even when a voice in my head says, "Endless browsing is not worthy of your time right now, go read a novel," twenty minutes go by, an hour, and I've been in thrall to the screen.

Sound familiar?

Nearly twenty years ago, my inner teachers began talking about all the changes that would be coming into our world. The positive side of it was that we would be awakening to our interconnectedness, we would be getting past what we'd been conditioned to think and feel, and we would develop clearer self-determination and agency.

We would be evolving to a new level of living and expression.

The negative side would be like what happens with food. It's appealing when we first prepare it and eat it, but it's significantly less lovely when the part we can't use comes out the other end! A friend of mine described the phenomenon of Mother Earth releasing what she no longer supports as "swamp gas." We have been experiencing lots of swamp gas for the last several years, seeing what happens as our collective body ejects what is not nutritious. We are smelling the ugliness of the world we are leaving behind up close and in stinky, vivid detail.

What I didn't anticipate in those moments when I was thrilled by the notion of evolving to a new level was how thoroughly the changes would destabilize most of us. How cultures around the world would polarize into rampant us-versus-them-ness. How it would play out in actual events. How we would feel insecure. And how the very nature of *truth* and *fact* and *reality* would come into question with loud voices claiming to know what other people should do.

I also didn't anticipate the phenomenon that *New York Times* bestselling author Rachel Maddow called "transgressive thrill," the pushing of boundaries and norms beyond their breaking point in an apparent frenzy to take down the system that somehow let you down. It reminds me of playing the card game Hearts as a kid. You don't want to get the Queen of Spades, because it gives you 26 points (and points are bad). But if you do get the Queen, the only way forward to win big is to capture all the hearts as well, and then you "shoot the moon" and everyone else gets the 26 points instead.

I somehow believed that the changes would only happen to people who hadn't been working on themselves, hadn't been trying to awaken, to cultivate their deeper truth. But I've come to see that we are *all* being asked to make structural and internal changes in how we live, work, relate to others, perceive events, use our energies, and make choices.

It is tempting to want to withdraw from the world, go back to a mythical better past, or jump in with crusading verve to save the planet. Instead, I think we each need to *at least* do our piece of it: adjust and evolve our instruments to play a different kind of music in different kinds of orchestras.

We need to help ourselves, and we need to help one another, to create a world that makes sense and has meaning.

● ● ●

I'm not gearing up here to dive into all the scary threats to our future that many of us see stalking our world right now. I'm inviting you instead to explore with me the question of how we can evolve our body-mind-spirit energies so we can have more agency in our lives, so we can play a more active role in creating ourselves, in co-writing shared narratives, and in co-creating the world we'd like to see.

My goal in this book is to share practical tools and insights on how to work with the mechanism in each of us that my inner teachers call the "Storymaker."

Your Storymaker is the mechanism that helps you create your "self."
It weaves energies into coherence to make meaning.

When I couldn't tell which tiger was real and felt myself blurring and my sense of reality dissolving as I fell down the rabbit hole, that was my Storymaker taking a hit, losing its balance, and becoming temporarily dysregulated. In that state, I lost perspective. I started spinning stories that made my sense of orientation even less stable. And I triggered panic in another energy mechanism that protects the self: my Gatekeeper.

Your Gatekeeper is the part of you that guards the gates of self. It manages your fight, flight, freeze, or fog reactivity and protection.

I remember vividly the first time I realized I had a Storymaker and how crucial and life-changing it would be for me to learn to work with it. It was in the late 1980s. I was in the habit of going twice a year to a silent meditation retreat, just to clear out my mind and rest it. I suffer from an ailment I have always called "sticky brain." Once I hear something, I have trouble letting it go. Once I see something, I have trouble unseeing it, especially if it is disturbing. And the details of that story, the emotions and nuances and emotional imperatives of it, will keep catching my attention long after I'm no longer being exposed to it.

I suspect it might be hereditary. My father had a photographic memory; my aunt on my mother's side, at ninety-eight, still remembers details of all the songs she learned and stories she has heard, even when it's about a neighbor's second cousin's new husband. My own sticky brain used to involve re-living conversations and re-seeing imagery that upset me. I already knew to avoid scary shows and looking at images of diseased skin. But I found it helped me manage my sticky brain to spend a week in silence, twice a year, just emptying the holding tanks.

So, at this particular meditation retreat, I was stuck in an endless loop of defending myself against my partner's ex, Louise. I kept trying to explain to her why she didn't need to hate me, why I wasn't a threat, why she could move on. And I wasn't just re-living the dozen or so moments when she was mean to me. Although I was doing my best to stay empty and present, I was spiraling into a whole new storyline in my head. Maybe she had powers, witchy powers, and could reach me and infect me energetically. Maybe she was actively invading my mind, even as I sat there trying to be open.

I kept breathing and kept observing the sticky brain working its dubious magic. And then I heard a voice in my head say, "It's not Louise. SHE'S NOT HERE."

Just like that, I realized that almost *all* my Louise pain, resistance, and storyline had been created inside me. I had written the Louise story! She was a walk-on, albeit a nasty one in real life, in a drama I was creating and perpetuating. If I wanted to be liberated, if I wanted to have a life of meaning, not at the mercy of the Louises in my life, I would have to learn to work with the part of me that created the stories.

Because the meditation put me in touch with the sensations arising and receding, I was equally clear in that moment that this was not just in my head. This story affected my physical body, my wiring, and my ability to feel healthy and well; it emanated from some part of me that selects the stories I think of as "my life." And, furthermore, I saw in that aha moment that the stories I was choosing were not ones chosen from my heart, or gut, or inner knowing. I could see them woven through me, energetic structures, reflecting earlier fear and prejudice and pain, limiting and creating my experience of being alive. And I could see that healing my sticky brain would require more than just emptying my mind at an occasional retreat. I needed to learn more about the parts of me creating and guarding the stories and how to help myself make different choices.

From that day on, that phrase "She's not here" became a touchstone for me. Whenever something is bothering me, getting me all bent out of shape, I remind myself, "She's not here." It pulls me out of my story, and then I can use energy medicine to reset my energies to support and respond to a different narrative.

Because I was more than ten years into being trained by my inner teachers at that point, I already carried a belief that we are creating ourselves from the inside out, that each of us chooses, over and over, what settings, character, plot, motivation, voice, and other aspects of our lived experience to register as our reality. When I say "choose," I don't mean "control." But we are each authoring and coauthoring all day long, and so the more conscious we can be of our storylines and how they influence us, the healthier we can be.

This was my first moment of seeing and feeling the mechanics of how this happens. It was like seeing the inside of a clock and realizing that "time" was not just an abstract; it was also something ticking away mechanically.

And because I saw, in that moment, that Louise was a walk-on in my drama and that most of what was bothering me about her was *not* interactive, it freed me to change the terms of engagement. The Louise I had created in my inner story quickly dropped away. And when I next saw the actual Louise, I just registered her presence and moved on. I let go of my end of the rope, and from then on, it was no longer such a troubling connection.

• • •

The Storymaker's job is to create frameworks and context to guide the energies we are made of. In particular, it manages patterns, integrates our different energy systems, and supports us in our creation of self. Here are a few of its defining features:

◆ It is built into every one of our energy systems.

◆ It helps us discern our own reality and truth.

◆ It serves the part of our being that craves and seeks meaning.

◆ It supports and helps us craft and stay true to narratives that align with our soul's priorities.

◆ It offers us an inner compass aligned with our inner true north.

◆ It enables us to find agency within our lived experience.

If you don't know what I mean by energy systems, don't worry. In coming chapters, you will learn what that means. But, for now, I will just say this: You are made of energies (though you appear solid). Your body, mind, and spirit communicate using energy. It is the language your body speaks, even though we are taught in our culture to think that the body communicates primarily via chemical signaling. And you can use energy communications to influence and participate in the workings of your body, mind, and spirit.

It is quite magical to discover that you can communicate with your own body, your own creation this way, and make a real difference in your health and well-being! In our shared Western medical beliefs, rooted in the body's chemistry and physical functions, energy is seen as exotic and maybe too foreign or woo-woo. But, in much of the world, energy medicine *is* the understanding of what is happening in your body, mind, and spirit and how to heal it.

To experience energy communication, try this simple energy exercise:

Exercise: Reconciliation

Call to mind a story that has been bothering you lately. It may be something personal, like an argument you had with a colleague; it might be something from a news article that is getting you down or making you feel life is not what you'd like it to be. You might want to give this story a title such as "What's Happening in the Middle East" or "What My Colleague and I Are Avoiding Right Now" or "My Persistent Stomach Issues."

Tune in to where in your body this story is affecting you and how it makes you feel physically, emotionally, energetically, and mentally. You may not know exactly where or how the story is affecting you, but it's good to gently touch various parts of your body to invite them into the conversation.

Keep the story in mind as you take these steps:

1. Rub your hands together to activate them to communicate.

2. Place one hand flat over your belly button (palm facing the belly button). Feel your palm and belly button making a connection.

3. Place your other hand flat on your back, directly behind your belly button. (If you can't reach, you can just use fingertips or lean against a balled-up cloth to activate this area of your back.) This area is called the Mingmen area in Eden Energy Medicine (also known as Eden Method), and it is a doorway to some of your deeper energies.

4. Now, send energy in a figure-eight pattern between your two hands, through your body, front to back, back to front, moving continuously. Feel the energy moving between your hands as you would feel the movement of a ball you are tossing from hand to hand.

Note: If you don't feel a figure-eight pattern moving between your hands, you can first trace figure eights front to back on each side of your body at the waist, getting a more felt sense of that figure-eighting motion and energy.

Then place your hands once again on your belly button and Mingmen point and send the energies figure-eighting front and back through your body.

5. Continue holding and "figure-eighting" (sending figure eights) until you sense a shift in your relationship to the story you are focused on. Often the energies will shift in about three minutes.

6. Tune in. What has altered for you, in your mind, feelings, and body sensations as you name or think of the story?

The purpose of this exercise isn't to remove the story from your brain. It is to reconcile your inner truth with the outer dimensions of the story coming at you from the world. Your subtle energies naturally travel in a figure-eight pattern, so sending figure eights this way supports your healthiest energy flow. Because your Mingmen area is a doorway to inner depths and knowing, and your belly button is the doorway to getting nourished from *out there* in the world, you can use this simple, loving energy communication to reconcile those two sources in you.

Energy communication is rich and varied. It offers many ways to work with both the Storymaker and the stories as they influence our bodies. It gives us access to influencing our stories as they form, as we live them, and as they affect our physical, emotional, mental, and spiritual well-being.

And that brings me to a key point of this book: *Your body lives your story.* It lives the truth you use to frame your experience. It lives the energy dynamics embedded in your understanding of what you are living.

This is not just some abstract concept. Imagine this: You are awakened in the night by a noise. It seems quite loud in the silence of your house. You think, *Oh no, someone is trying to break in!* Immediately your heartbeat quickens and your breathing gets shallow. You feel adrenaline coursing through your body, and you start to shake. You try to push back your rising panic. You have set the story and your body is living it.

What should I do? You reach out for your phone, then remember that you left it in the bathroom, about fourteen feet away. You wonder, *Can I get there quietly without alerting the intruder?*

You start imagining scenarios. You think you might hear creaking on the stairs. *Is the intruder coming upstairs?* Can you somehow surprise and over-power him, using the martial arts moves you've seen on TV? Can you hit him with your lamp? As you think this, you feel your muscles bunching and tightening, as if already practicing.

You try to quietly wake up the person sleeping next to you to confer: *What should we do?* But they are breathing smoothly and easily. You try a gentle touch to wake them without causing an outcry. They just roll over and breathe deeply.

Unbeknownst to you, your companion also woke up when something went bump in the night. But they thought, *It's the cat jumping onto her favorite perch.* And smiling slightly, feeling love and warmth at the image, your companion settled into an even more relaxed and contented rhythm of breathing. They feel your gentle touch as confirmation: *That was our sweet kitty.*

Now, it's completely silent. You are pretty sure there are no more creaking noises on the stairs. And nothing seems to be moving downstairs. You don't quite feel ready to go down and investigate. Maybe you do creep into the bathroom to grab your phone to keep it near you in case you need to call for help. And you lie there for at least an hour, wide-awake, listening intently, muscles tight, breathing shallow, on alert for any more indications of a presence, until finally, exhaustion takes over and you fall asleep.

In this way, your body lives your stories. Every thought, every image, and every situation registers on your body chemically and energetically, affecting your breathing, digestion, muscle tone, alignment of your bones, tissue break-down and buildup, and more.

This link between story and body is more than just the release of adrenaline when you are scared. It happens at each moment you draw breath, each time you have an experience. In your mind, interpretation and storymaking are happening. In your body, chemical and physiological adaptations are happening, and what's happening in your mind and body are happening in response to each other. Often these thoughts, images, situations, and body reactions also give rise to feelings meant to help you steer the ship. These feelings both color and reflect your story.

You may have heard people claim that our thoughts create our reality or that our beliefs call in our experiences or that feelings are our guide to truth. And while these are each true to an extent, there is something more going on. It is this something more we will explore in the coming chapters.

This book is designed to be used in a variety of ways:

1. You can read straight through, treating the exercises and sections called "Play with It!" as additional dimensions to the discussion. Then, you can return later to try the exercises and activities that call to you.

2. You can stop reading periodically to try the explorations and exercises. You may be surprised at what you experience in terms of your own personal evolution. The activities are designed to be individualized, to help you co-write this path of awakening with me—not to lead you to certain conclusions I may have found. I believe we each have inner guidance and our own unique gifts. Let yourself dance with the energy concepts and information in this book on your own terms.

3. You can use this book as a course book to help you broaden and deepen your study of energy medicine.

4. If you aren't linear, you can use this book as a divination tool. Ask for insight into something, and open the book to wherever you are drawn. Let that topic or the stories or activities you find there animate your own knowing.

My goal is for this book to help you get to know your own Storymaker in ways that make sense and have meaning for you! In the end, I hope each person who reads this book hears their own inner truth and guidance a bit more clearly.

If you have read my earlier work, a handful of exercises in this book may already be familiar to you. I've brought them back here to expand, extend, or show how they can be used to dialogue with your Storymaker. If you are the kind of person who always wants to learn new techniques, I encourage you to explore how you can also use familiar tools in new ways.

Feel free to adapt the energy medicine exercises, protocols, guided visits, and Play with Its! to your own speed and style. If you like quick spontaneous explorations, just step in and try them. If you are someone who needs to get centered or prefers to explore energy in a slower, more contemplative state, use whatever tools work for you (breathing, meditation, journaling, etc.) to get yourself into your preferred rhythm. Since this work is about communicating with your own energies, you can experiment with what works best for you.

A NOTE ABOUT TERMINOLOGY

Many wise healers and teachers have taught about energy for thousands of years. There are energy features that most of us have heard of, such as chakras and auras and meridians. I want to honor that body of tradition and knowledge. But, at the same time, my inner teachers often use their own terminology, perhaps to keep me from falling into the trap of thinking I truly understand phenomena that I am merely familiar with in my brain. So, if the terms "Storymaker" or "Gatekeeper" don't resonate with you, find your own names for these mechanisms. Maybe one of the most important aspects of reclaiming our agency is our willingness to choose the names and labels that work best for us.

If you find yourself straining to see how this work fits other modalities you have studied, take a moment to step back and ask instead, "How do these concepts and practices fit with my understanding of my own lived experiences? How can I use this material to tune my instrument and figure out new ways to play it?"

I have come to believe that healing your story is a crucial part of physical healing. It is by necessity a deeply personal quest. But working with these lesser-known energy mechanisms is also key to healing our shared lives and our world. In this time of overwhelming information overload, I think it has become crucial for us to learn how to keep our Storymakers healthy and strong, discern our own truth, clear out old stories that don't serve us, and evolve our mind-body to create a more authentic life.

• • •

If you have purchased this book or received it as a gift and would like help with the guided visits and exercises, visit EllenMeredith.com/storyline for downloadable MP3s and links to videos. Please enter your name and email address and use the password cominghome.

CHAPTER ONE

Listen and Learn

The baby, she said, was due any time now. And he was breech. Her doctor was threatening she'd need a risky procedure to turn the baby if he didn't turn by tomorrow. Could I do anything to help? Sandra was calling me from her doctor's office in a panic. "I don't want to force him. Can't you tune in to see what's going on?"

It was 1984, and I'd been introduced to Sandra as "a psychic" a month or so earlier by her chiropractor, Barbara, when I began my accidental career in her office, using my intuitive abilities as a consultant with patients who needed insight into what was happening with their healing. The DA after my name, while an actual doctorate, stood for doctor of arts, not doctor of anything medical.

This was my first request to see someone for healing work outside the protective shield of that office. "Can we meet at Barbara's?" I asked, thinking, *I know nothing, absolutely nothing, about birthing babies.*

"She doesn't have any openings until next Friday."

A voice in my head, my inner teachers, who I call my Councils, said, "Listen and learn. You won't know if you don't try."

"Well," I said, "I don't know anything about childbirth, but if you want to come over, I'll tune in and see what the baby has to say." She said she'd be right over.

I wandered into the other room. This was long before Google, so I couldn't quickly look up childbirth. Instead, I told Orla, the woman I lived with at the time, what had just happened. Since she was an MD in family practice, I asked if she had any advice or cautions.

"Oh, fun! Can I come too?" she asked.

An hour later, with Sandra's permission, Orla was examining her to verify the baby was indeed breech. He was—apparently, spectacularly so. They both looked expectantly at me: *Now what?* And that's when my lessons in being willing to listen and learn kicked in. At that point, I'd been training intensively with my Councils for about seven years. They had predicted that after I moved to California, I'd learn to be a healer—was this it?

I put my hands on both sides of Sandra's huge belly, about where the baby's head and feet were, and opened up to hearing what this little being wanted and needed. He wasn't talking to me in words. I just got a sense that he was feeling uninterested in moving from this safe, warm space. I could feel his mother's anxiety, but he was used to that and was ignoring it.

Hmmm, I thought, *what are the ethics of trying to talk this baby into getting a move on? Maybe he just needs to cook a little longer.* I tried to ask him mentally, "Do you need more time?" He had no idea what I was asking. I realized that he was stuck in his "now." He had no sense of himself in a transition, from womb to living outside the womb. He was comfortable and utterly without ambition and had no picture of anything else.

I asked my Councils, *Now what?*

They said, "Listen to your hands."

While I was sitting there trying to figure this out with my brain, my hands had been warming up and were in deep dialogue with both the baby and the mother's womb. I saw and felt, emanating from my hands, the family he was being born into, his two loving moms, the sense of fun and laughter they wanted to teach him, the journey they had gone through to come together and conceive him, first in their hearts and minds, and then, in Sandra's womb. He was a donor insemination baby, and I could feel the energy of the donor there too, cheering from the sidelines. And then I felt the extended families and clans he was being born into and had come from, the affiliations this soul had formed through many lifetimes.

As I sank my attention into this larger perception of his being, I felt some movements. Not kicking exactly. Undulations. He was *swimming* into the birth position! I just held the space and my hands continued to communicate, cheering him on. And then the movement stopped. I felt the warmth recede, felt him settle into his new state.

I looked at Sandra and Orla and said, "I think he turned." Orla confirmed it.

We all sat there grinning at one another, until Sandra said, "Well, thanks. Can you be with me at the birth?"

Oh no!

I heard my Councils say again, "Listen and learn."

"Okay," I said. "Just call when it's time."

About four days later, I was at the lovely, homey, newly renovated birthing center of the local hospital with Sandra and her partner. I was panicking once again, because I still didn't know anything about birthing babies. Sandra was having contractions and not happy with the pain. She was particularly worried about her newly healed back and neck, which had brought her to the chiropractor's office where we met. I thought I might be there as a kind of insurance policy, since I'd been able to readjust her bones at the office, using energy when physical manipulation wouldn't work.

Sandra was anxious but also determined to be fully present for the birth, not wanting an epidural or other pain meds. After several hours of watching her spasm with pain, I thought, *If this was me, I'd be going for the drugs by now.* I was doing what I could to just be there as support and witness, for both her and her partner.

But, at some point, the doctor bustled in, checked her dilation and monitors, and said, "Things aren't progressing the way they should. The baby is getting agitated." (They had a monitor on his heart too.) "If things don't move soon, we're going to need to induce you."

When she bustled out, Sandra turned to me in a panic. "Can't you do something?"

Oh, god, I thought, *this is it: I'm about to be outed as a charlatan!*

I *really* didn't know what I was doing there. I looked away for a second, trying to figure out how I could support her. And, in the corner of the room, I saw a woman—well, a spirit—who said, "I'll show you how to do this." She was Filipino, looked to be in her sixties, and said, "I'm Josefina. I'm a midwife."

Hallelujah! Score one for the Universe.

Josefina said, "She needs to open gradually. She is trying to just open up completely all at once and let the baby out, but her body is fighting this.

Instead, ask her to picture her womb as a set of nested drawstring bags. When I give the signal, you will touch her belly where she needs to direct her attention, and with her exhales, she will open the drawstring of that one, particular bag."

With great relief, I explained this to Sandra, and about a minute later, Josefina showed me where the first bag needed to open. Sandra's partner and I both mirrored her with long, powerful exhales. And I kept my hand on the opening for that bag until I felt the drawstring release and the bag slide open.

For the next hour, Sandra was too busy opening the bags and resting in between to continue to angst about her ability to do this. Her doctor bustled in, checked the monitor, and told us that the baby's heartbeat was now normal. She said, "Things are progressing finally; you are dilating at a good pace."

We didn't tell her about the drawstring bags, but we could all three feel them—the ones that were already open and the ones still needing to be released.

I don't have a sense of how long it took to get all the bags opened—but, after the first few, Sandra had learned to work with the process and was no longer screaming in pain. She was becoming more focused and turning inward, and Josefina continued to not only show us the next bag but also gave little tips on where Sandra's body needed support: to be held, a little pressure or pulsing, to be anchored by her partner, or the two of us working together to help her ride the waves moving her baby into the birth canal.

When it came time to push, she was fully inside the process, and it took only about fifteen minutes for her nine-pound, eight-ounce bruiser to be born.

I turned to thank Josefina, but she was already gone. The story doesn't end there, though.

Some weeks later, Orla returned from, of all places, a trip to the Philippines. She was interested in learning more about different healing modalities and had spent a month traveling around the countryside, visiting faith healers and other traditional healers. I told her about our spirit, Josefina, showing up to coach the birth. Orla got a strange look on her face, excused herself, left the room for a few minutes, and returned with a sheaf of brochures. She lined them up, with the photos of each healer she had contacted sitting side by side like a police lineup, and said, "Recognize anybody?"

There she was: the third photo from the left—Josefina! It was clearly the same person. And far from being a spirit of a dead person, she was very much still alive, practicing as a midwife and traditional healer in a remote area of the Philippines. Orla had tried to visit her but was told she was off on retreat. (I heard she died about a year later.)

This was still relatively early in my getting to know the World Wise Web (the original *www*). I heard the theme music from *The Twilight Zone* playing in my head. We speculated for a while about how Josefina knew to show up and the coincidence (synchronicity) of her touching *both* our lives around the same time, and we marveled over the brilliance of her drawstring bag strategy.

That evening as I lay in bed, a time when I often felt more open to guidance, Josefina showed up again in my mind. She said, "I'd like to introduce you to a group called the Tibetans. It is a group of healers your Wiser Self has belonged to for some time." (*Wiser Self* was the term my Councils used for the part of us that is part of the Divine, and lives in the realm of soul and spirit.)

I found myself at a long table, where a group of souls who she described as healers from all over the world, from many cultures and times, were meeting. They offered me a seat at the table. They said, "Some of us are *in body*, meeting here, as you are meeting us here. Others are *in spirit.* We are working to bring healing to the world. We invite you to join with us. We meet here as needed to support our joint vision to teach healing to people and cultures that need it. And we often share techniques, as Josefina did with you."

I wondered why they were called Tibetans. Clearly hearing my thoughts, they said, "Our spiritual roots grew from that place, but we span the globe and beyond." Needless to say, I accepted their invitation to join their group. And, as my Councils had predicted, I was on my path to becoming a healer.

Fast forward to the mid-2020s, and this story is on my mind a lot lately. It was the set of events that made me realize that while skepticism is healthy and useful, there is clearly more to reality than my Michigan-grown brain thought. It was the time in my personal life when I was brought to experience what author Joseph Chilton Pearce dubbed "the crack in the cosmic egg"—the breaking apart of logic and rationality to understand that there is more to reality and the life force than meets the eye.

This story is up for me now because we are again entering a time when the old ways of seeing and knowing and organizing ourselves are breaking apart. And a new world is being born. For many of us, it is painful, and we are trying to open fully, but our bodies and minds are fighting it. And I'm thinking that Josefina was on to something: If we can work with change the way Sandra worked with her drawstring bags, maybe we can enter into it, rather than being swept away by the discomfort. If we can locate where in our bodies, our lives, and our minds the opening needs to take place—where the drawstring needs to be released—we might be able to avoid numbing drugs such as news addiction and binge-watching and stay present for the new being we are birthing.

Like thousands of other psychic channels, healers, seers, and prognosticators all over the world, I see this as a time when the old ways (hopefully the patriarchy) are dying and new ways (hopefully more compassionate, humane, and powered from within) are being born. But if we don't want to mangle the baby, we all need to know a bit more about how to listen and learn.

Here's what my Councils had to say about this time:

One of the themes of this time you are living is the breaking apart of myths, of beliefs about how life works and should work. Each of you will be finding yourself questioning the mores, the ways things are done, the norms. These narratives—about how life is and should be—have historically offered frameworks to guide collective and individual behaviors. But, in this time of great transformation, you will each need to become myth busters and creators of new stories. You will be learning greater discernment and will awaken not only to what is untrue and limiting in the shared reality but also to what your deep inner truth can contribute to a new kind of shared reality.

What do we each need so we can work with this cosmic wave of contraction and expansion?

First, we need to *access our own experiences*. We need to be able to hear the echoes and guidance of our deep inner truth within our own stories and our own reality as we live it.

Second, we need to *tune in to what within us needs to be born* and find ways, if necessary, to help it swim into position and bring it safely through a birth canal that will allow it passage.

Third, we need to be able to **break down the process so it's tolerable** in order to participate in it and not get overwhelmed.

Fourth, we need to learn how to **support our bodies through the stress** of everyday personal transformation and massive worldly change.

Fifth, we need to **access the World Wise Web**, the inner and outer community of individuals and groups working to co-create what we'd like to be part of. For me, that is a world that celebrates and is enriched by a person's gifts. It's a world where compassion is normal and power comes in the form of empowerment, not power over. And it's a world where power is understood as motive force, not as something wrested from the earth and that pollutes our air. That's my personal wish list. What's yours?

Sixth, we need to **become creators**, giving birth to and parenting this new world to fulfill its potential. We need to gain agency within ourselves by opening to the inner worlds that fuel and connect us. That awareness can guide us if we are willing to listen and learn how to navigate in this strange new world that is evolving faster than we ever imagined.

|||||||||||||| **Play with It!** ||||||||||||||

Josephina's drawstring bags can help you open up your head, your heart, your gut, or any part of your being where a process is painful and not progressing. It is not limited to the womb.

Take a moment to think of a situation where you feel tight, constricted, and unable to move forward or back.

If the situation is physical, you will work in that area of your body (or work symbolically on that area of your body if it is a place you can't reach). If the situation is in your mind, emotions, work, relationship, or somewhere out there, ask that situation to appear in front of you as an image. You don't need to actually see the image. You will interact with it as if you can see it.

Now, tune in and let your attention be called to the first drawstring bag that needs to be opened. (If you are adventuresome, invite Josefina or another healer in to coach you.)

Take a deep breath in, and on the exhale, use your hands to loosen the drawstring and open that bag. This works much better if you use your hands and gesture to mime opening the bag. If you usually do exercises using visualization, I strongly encourage you to break free from that habit and try using gesture with your imagery. Gesture helps pull the experience into your full body, away from your sometimes overly trained brain.*

Once you have opened, smoothed, and where appropriate, pulled the first bag away from the area, tune in to what you are experiencing as a result of this action. You can always explore the bag itself, as well as the liberated inner bundle.

Here's an example:

> I have been experiencing severe eyestrain lately and pressure in my eyeballs (glaucoma). My first bag, I intuit, surrounds my whole head. I open the drawstring, which is tight around my neck, and on the exhale, I smooth the bag, pull it up off my head, and remove it. As I do this, I feel a level of tension release, and a mild headache eases. I remove at least three nested bags here before I feel pulled to a different area.

If the baby is nearing its time to be born, you will want to continue to open each bag, adjust to the new state, breathe, and wait until you sense it is time to open the next bag. If you are just exploring what all is enclosed in your nested bags, you might open one bag at a time and investigate: What was that bag, that restriction, holding you in place? Give yourself time to really feel and get used to the liberation of opening the drawstring.

---

* For me, gesture works well. But if you are literal-minded, you can actually assemble a set of nested drawstring bags, place a piece of paper with the name of the issue or situation you are trying to open (or some kind of image or symbolic representation) in the innermost bag, then when doing this, you will literally open one bag at a time, get it good and open, clear the wrinkles, and pull it away from the nested bundle.

When you are ready, let your inner Josefina show you which bag comes next. Take a deep breath, and on the exhale, mime opening the bag. Feel how easy or challenging this is, how tight or loose the drawstring was. If there is a knot, you may need to get creative to untangle it.

Take time to listen and learn, and jot down what you are experiencing with each bag. You may not understand it right away. Tune in to what it feels like and what, if anything, shifts within you when you loosen the drawstring. Sometimes, you will have an immediate release. But often the change takes twenty-four hours or more to grow into something you can sense and know. Give yourself time to really explore this opening, rather than focusing on getting the baby out asap.

Continuing with my example:

My next bag surrounds my left eye. As I release it, I feel my eyeball fluttering, like a newly hatched butterfly drying its wings. I shut my eyes to feel it gain strength and eventually take flight.

My next bag is around my right eye. It is sticky and difficult to move the material over the string. It feels as if the string is tangled inside the cloth. I keep hearing, "I don't want to see! This world is crazy. Don't want that energy in my brain." I coat my glasses with an energy filter keyed to act like a holding tank that gives me time to take things in. It gives me space between my brain and the world it is seeing. Then the protests quiet down.

I notice a bag around my entire face. This one has drawstrings both top and bottom. So it is more like a sleeve than a bag. When I pull it off, I feel a release in the muscles of my face, including my jaw muscles.

Although I sense more bags (for example, around the ears), I decide to stop and get used to this new state.

Each time you use this technique, you are likely to have a different experience. This is meant to facilitate birthing, but understand, not all babies are ready to be born! As you do this, listen and learn what the challenge is asking of you, what it needs, and what you need to bring in new life.

ACCESS YOUR INNER TRUTH

Josefina nailed it when she said, "She needs to open gradually." Sandra was tangled up and blocked because she was pushing herself to open, and her body and mind fought back. When she had a method for taking it one bag at a time, she was able to tolerate and participate in the process.

I always hesitate to tell the more woo-woo stories about my training with my Councils because people say, "That's just you, you're psychic." But I believe, and my experience backs me up, that we are all psychic. We are each born with the ability to hear inner truth, to know things from our inner affiliations and larger nature, and to activate reliable inner guidance; it is built into the mind-body instrument. I find it sad that we live in a culture with such a distorted understanding of this glorious instrument that many of us believe we can't access our inner knowing.

That's a myth we need to bust now. And, with that, we need workable techniques to explore our inner byways and learn from reliable sources, so we don't just replace our former knowing or beliefs with someone else's revealed truth. Beware of those spiritual paths that tell you how the inner worlds are structured and what you should find there. And beware of the "hacks" designed to get you to the goal without experiencing a journey. (I assume you know to beware of social media groupthink!)

Wisdom is more than a chemical state in the brain. It's more than feeling awake in a way that makes your adrenaline run. It's even more than the euphoria and high of transcendence. It's what arises when we create our own understandings of life from the inside out and forge an instrument that allows us to both support our own unique nature and contribute to the larger good.

Another myth that floats around spiritual communities is that the path to inner awakening is meditation, meditation, and more meditation. If you are one of those people who just can't meditate, this is quite a roadblock. Don't get me wrong—I love meditation and find it useful to clear my mind and enter silence. But I also know that if you believe you can only hear your truth in the emptiness, you miss the fact that your inner world is constantly broadcasting the fullness of your larger being and the music of your soul.

To say it in a less poetic way: Your inner world is communicating with you constantly, even reflecting back at you from events outside yourself. It is a language that is your birthright, and you can relearn it by letting yourself take it one step at a time.

It's not a linear process, so you're not going to get grammar lessons here. Instead, it's a process of engaging inward over and over again to listen (see, feel, smell, taste, know) and learn. It's a process of being in a relationship, a love affair, with your own inner byways.

ALL IN YOUR MIND

I recently asked a class of spiritual seekers, "Where is your mind?" Most of them pointed to their heads, drawing a kind of aura or halo around the head to indicate it was in a space occupied by, but somewhat bigger than, their brain. That is a common way to frame understanding of the mind.

But a key skill in opening to spiritual wisdom, in getting beyond the trained brain, is a willingness to try *reframes*. A reframe is what it sounds like: You take the story or belief you are telling yourself about something (even if it's something most people believe), and you put a frame or shape around it that shifts your perspective *and* your ability to grow.

You might say, "Taylor Swift has problems with relationships," because she writes song after song about her love woes. This is a judgment on poor Taylor and doesn't get you very far. But you can also frame it differently: "Taylor Swift has a lot to teach us about relationships because she's explored many of them, and she distills her learning so articulately to share with us."

Which frame is going to allow Taylor to thrive and allow you to learn from her?

If you find yourself believing something like "The mind resides in and around your head," ask yourself if that concept of the mind is large enough, true enough. Does it support you to evolve and thrive? Or do you find yourself stuck in your head with nowhere to go?

I like to look to our spoken language to see if other views emerge from folk wisdom to shed light on the belief in question—for example, *I know it in my bones . . . in my heart, in my gut, down to my toes, in my blood, down to my soul, through and through.* Our grandmothers knew in these ways. We can too.

So, if I frame mind as being woven into every part of me—from soul to bones to gut, heart, and head, through and through—then getting to know and find knowing in my mind becomes a different task than if it's somehow a ghostly echo of my brain. I find it a relief to think of my mind this way. It means that when I "think," I can learn from how my gut and blood and toes and soul and every fiber of my being perceive and experience life.

TAKING SOUNDINGS

My favorite way to cultivate this whole mind kind of perception is what I call "taking soundings." It is an ongoing practice of tuning in to various parts of my mind (every fiber of my being), not just to answer questions, but to cultivate input on what my whole being is experiencing.

When something is bothering me—say I've got a health decision to make, or I have to decide which of the too many things on my agenda can be dropped, or just when I want to know my own inner truth about something—I take soundings. I let my whole mind weigh in and show me. I also, of course, listen in at each place for guidance.

The goal of taking soundings is to get past your trained brain to hear knowing from within. Here's how it works:

1. Ask open-ended questions or just open up to perceive what is there.

An open-ended question is one that generates possibilities and insights. Here are some examples:

- ◆ "Give me insight into . . . "

- ◆ "What can you tell me about . . . ?"

- ◆ "Where might this choice lead me?"

- ◆ "What do I need to recognize about . . . ?"

- ◆ "What territory does this choice inhabit?"

While not technically framed as a question, "Give me insight into . . ." is my favorite way of easing into a conversation with my mind. This is because yes-no questions can sometimes confuse the body. If you ask, "Should I go to the dance?" the body doesn't know what aspect of the experience you are asking about. The physical experience of dancing? The social implications of showing up? The time you'd spend or waste if you went? If you ask, "Give me insight into my choice of going to the dance," your mind and body can respond with how that choice would affect each of them. And, of course, you can then specify: "Give me insight in how going to the dance might affect my physical fatigue," or "Give me insight into my emotions about going to the dance."

Our culture just *loves* right/wrong, yes/no answers (or multiple-choice answers). Should I get that surgery? Do I need to quit my job? Is this the right path for me? That love of clarity papers over the fact that very few, if any, situations are cut-and-dried. Even if you ultimately choose one over the other, there is the more nuanced question of how you live that choice and what you give up by making it.

When we look for right answers, we often miss the guidance and insights we are getting.

Pam had a deep desire to develop her intuition and hear what her Wiser Self had to say to her. She took a number of classes offering exercises meant to help her explore her inner byways. However, each time she did an exercise to get insight, she'd get restless, sometimes itchy, and her mind would jump in to argue with the process: *How do I know that's true? What does that really mean? Am I just making this up?* She'd be up in her head, all tangled in obsessive thoughts.

When this happened to her during an exploration of taking soundings, I asked her, "What question did you ask?"

She said, "What I always ask: What is blocking me from hearing my inner truth?"

"And what happened," I asked, "when you did the exercise?"

She said, "What always happens: I got restless and jumpy. I couldn't sit still. In fact, I had to get up and walk around. And my mind started in with questions about why I couldn't do this. What was wrong with me. Whether I had the wrong question."

"Well," I said, "it looks to me like your body answered the question beautifully. It *showed* you your blockage. What blocks you is believing you should sit still. Try moving and dancing your insights."

Pam looked confused for a moment, and then it sank in. She put both hands on her heart and nodded, with a look of relief on her face.

I went on, "And fear is coming up. Often that arises because in this life or another you've died—as a witch, a wise woman, a seer, an iconoclast—because of this knowing. So your body is asking you to clear some of those templates and to recognize you are taking too much on at once. Instead of asking what is blocking you, ask what would support you. Instead of asking for 'inner truth,' how about asking for input into a more manageable question such as 'Give me insight into what might enrich my evening.'" (See chapter 8 for more on templates.)

Pam had been trying to open all the drawstring bags at once, and I saw her relax when she realized she could approach her habitual question in terms of what might work moment by moment, rather than asking for an all-inclusive explanation of her blockage.

"Finally," I said, "your body showed you how your mind loves to dominate and think itself through a situation, question the givens. Brain thinking is what we are taught to do in our culture, and questioning the authority of the question is a healthy impulse. But that can block other ways of knowing. Why not try to include your brain in the conversation? Do some free writing ahead of time to *interview your brain*. Then, at each place you take the sounding, invite your brain to write a poem or song to capture what you experience there . . . or just to annotate with commentary. You can always analyze again later or dump the commentary."

The simple reframe from "I never can do this exercise" to "You've been given a response to what you asked" freed Pam to work with the information and start opening one bag at a time.

2. Gather information.

Our culture loves to interview and survey and come up with numerical assessments as a way to gather data. The problem with that is, usually the interview questions predetermine the direction of the conversation. And a survey ("Who thinks I should break up with Jordan?") often jumps to the attitudes, opinions, beliefs, and actions and skips over how that question affects all parts of you. It begs the question of what it means to be together with Jordan, and it mushes all the options into a binary: together/break up.

> *When you take soundings, you are not interviewing the parts of your mind; you are listening in and learning from what you find there.*

Similarly, we live in an impatient culture. We want the answer, and we want to know it now. That may be why the internet is so addictive. I look up *x* or *y*, and find what others have to say on the topic. Even when I trust the source, I am still jumping ahead to find the answer before I know if I'm even asking the right questions, before I understand the context, the dimensions, or the energetic truth of what I want to know and why.

So often, I've had students like Pam tune in to ask their body questions, only to say that they aren't getting an answer. That's because they are looking for an answer in their head, and they are not listening to hear (feel, smell, taste, see, and/or know) what is happening *energetically* in response to their question. Their mind wants the yes/no certainty of an answer, rather than gathering data, input to flavor the stew. I can identify with wanting certainty, but it will block your ability to hear in new ways in cases where your inner wisdom doesn't match your trained brain.

It is important to be patient, to be willing to not understand what you are perceiving or getting, and to learn over time what it means to you. It's not wrong to understand something right away. But if we want to get beyond our conditioned thinking, we need to leave space for not knowing, not understanding, and letting the new input teach us.

I find it useful to see the process of taking soundings as finding pieces to a jigsaw puzzle. You're going to put it together later, but first you have to pull all the pieces out of the box and organize them in front of you, so you can sort them and begin your assembly.

Here are two important aspects of taking soundings to gather information:

➤ Let information come to you in the language of energy, rather than expecting it to come full blown into your mind as words. This means you will use all your senses:

- Listen for sounds, rhythms, words, phrases, and voices.

- Look for imagery, colors, shapes, and patterns.

- Feel into both the sensations in your body and inner byways.

- Tune in to see if smell, taste, or texture arises.

- Perceive movement or stillness, flow, or blockage (or states in between).

- See if a gesture arises to express what you are picking up.

- Let direct knowing arise for you or ask for metaphors.

- Invite information about what is there and also what is not there (but is needed).

- Check to see if there are shifts or changes happening or being asked for.

- Recognize what you perceive in this place relative to cycles of buildup, fullness, release, and emptiness.

- See if you are connecting with guides in this place.

Note: I usually suggest waiting to seek guidance until you've listened and learned more directly using the language of energy. It is an art form to distinguish inner guidance from thoughts inserted by the trained brain trying to hang on to its reality. But you may get an image or phrase or knowing that you sense comes from a wise source. Gather it: You will assess it later.

➤ Let different aspects of yourself weigh in. You might get very different perspectives on a question from your feet, heart, or ears. And if you ask your child self, your future self, your Wiser Self, your professional self, or your private self, they too may have different perspectives to share.

Remember, the goal in taking soundings is to practice listening with your whole mind, your whole self, not just hearing your trained brain weigh in with thoughts.

3. Test your data as you interpret and put the puzzle pieces together.

It is tempting to get an insight and just run with it. But it's important to test what you are getting and explore whether it is metaphor or literal truth. Explore whether it fits with what you know or can verify in other ways. My Councils always encouraged me to work with their guidance this way, rather than just accepting everything they said (or I heard) as some kind of divine truth.

Brenda learned this lesson the hard way. She was learning to use her intuition and listen to inner guidance and was a bit obsessed with it. She kept saying to friends in a knowing tone of voice, "I've been told . . ." or "I see that you are. . . ." Most of her friends did not appreciate this because she was using this newfound source of information to win arguments or to be more right, and often she did not ask if her friends *wanted* her channeled guidance or insights. In other words, she was treating her evolving intuition as a commodity to bolster her ego rather than as a learning tool.

However, as often happens, the Universe stepped in. One morning, after she'd had a one-night stand where the condom failed, she tuned in to ask her inner guidance, "Am I pregnant?" She heard a clear answer: "Yes, you are pregnant." In a panic, she called up the man to tell him they were expecting a baby. She went into an emotional tailspin about how this baby would change her life. She spoke to several of her friends, who kept asking, "Are you sure?" She said, "Yes, I'm sure." And her life was in tumult for about ten days, until she got her period.

She felt betrayed by her inner guides and her body. How had this happened? Quite simply: The body and inner guides often speak and think in metaphors. Metaphorically, Brenda was cultivating new life, giving birth to new ways of understanding the world. She was pregnant with possibility. But she was not physically pregnant.

If she had understood that she needed to work with the information, test it against other sources of knowing, she could have waited to get a pregnancy test. She could have asked the follow-up questions: "Is this a fertilized egg implanted in my womb or a metaphoric truth?" If she hadn't been giving her intuition authority over her logic, she might have realized that it takes several days for a fertilized egg to implant and become a pregnancy. And if she had been willing to sit with the guidance, take it beyond yes/no questions, she might have gotten enough information to form a better understanding of the truth.

We can't always test everything objectively. But we can find other, additional ways to get information and give ourselves time and space to know more fully. I am a big believer that we should learn from the dialogues we have with our inner realms and evolve our intelligence to be both grounded and able to fly, to work with the box, even while we are trying to think outside it.

Exercise: Taking Soundings

As preparation, sit quietly and take a few deep breaths. Or do the Coming Home exercise on page 46.

1. Ask an open-ended question ("Give me insight into . . .") or just show up to tune in to each place where you want to take a sounding. Most soundings come quickly, so experiment with staying about ten to thirty seconds at each location. But if you are someone whose pace is naturally slower, adjust this activity to work for you.

2. Explore what you hear or perceive in response to your question as you place either hand on various parts of your body to take in what they have to communicate: What does each part of you contribute in terms of insight, need, yearning, and/or awareness? You are "listening" for images, sounds or words or songs, sensations, feelings, metaphors, imagined scenes, gestures, tastes, smells, direct knowing . . . even silence or blankness.

Keep your question in mind as you touch each body part in turn, taking a sounding at:

➤ Your elbows (separately or together)

➤ Your knees (separately or together)

➤ Your feet (separately or together)

➤ Your tailbone

➤ Your solar plexus

➤ Your sacral chakra (between your pubic bone and belly button)

➤ Your heart

➤ Your face

➤ Your ears

Feel free to take soundings in other places. Every part of your body can be a fruitful source of insight. Also, if you wish, ask your selves at various ages, your Wiser Self, and your future self to weigh in. Jot down what you receive with each sounding.

Tip: Don't overthink it. Whatever comes quickly is fine for now. You can return later to commune more deeply. Approach each sounding with curiosity and a sense of play. Don't try to make sense of what you get, just gather what shows up for you.

3. When you are done taking soundings, thank all the parts of you for their input. Take a look at what you picked up. You may understand clearly what you're being shown, or it may seem like a string of irrelevant images and sensations.

4. Sit with the information for at least forty-eight hours to build a fuller understanding of what you've perceived. Sometimes it takes a while to connect the dots and understand the message. You can always do some writing or talk it through with a close friend, who might be able to see the relevance your mind has not yet recognized.

Intuition that comes as a full package is often distorted by the mind that hears what it expects to hear. That's why taking soundings is so helpful. But because it is easy, remember this isn't your only chance to get insight. I often take soundings using the same question (or around the same issue) repeatedly over several days. That's because my mind will work with what it has given me and show me in other ways what I am not yet ready to know consciously.

If you get an unexpected thunderbolt insight or intuition or message, don't forget to question it. Test it out. Explore whether it is metaphoric or literal truth. Sit with it. Your body and mind need time to adjust to new frameworks, perspectives, and changing understandings of truth.

INNER GUIDANCE

Let's face it, most of us want a right-answer machine. We want an all-knowing inner or outer guru who can guide us in doubtful situations. When we are lucky, we find teachers—within us or outside us—who help us arrive at our own wisdom. When we are less lucky, we assign the role of guide to people or groups that aren't worthy of the power we give them.

The yearning to know who you are, how you are constructed, what your mission or purpose is, and who you share that mission with is something I suspect most of us feel. And it's my belief that the more we seek guidance within and ground it in our own unique being, including our stories of who and what we are, the more relevant and safe it will be.

Wars have been fought over the teachings of various prophets and seers. Whose truth is truthier? And like during the times of Jesus and the Buddha, there seems to be a lot of people claiming guru and Christ status these days. With the advent of our newest technologies (internet, social media, AI, 24/7 news outlets owned by special interests, etc.), power wars over the hearts and minds of the masses have been amplified and sent into overdrive. This is not a political statement: It is an observation of what is going on energetically in our world.

I believe the antidote, the solution, is for each of us to step up and find our own inner gifts. Not so we can compete for ascendancy and be more right, but so we can collaborate and work jointly on creating new social frameworks.

My work with the Tibetans taught me a lot about how such sharing and collaboration could work across the borders of time and space. From my perspective, it was cool and woo-woo, and something I have not talked about before, even with close friends and mentors. Now that we have video chat and internet, those kinds of collaborations, at least the kind that happen among people in bodies who share creative solutions and teachings from the past, can come into being without so much woo.

As far as I know, wars have not been fought over our inner teachers, our individual sources of inspiration and soul juice. So I believe the time is more than ripe for us each to develop inner guidance and soul-level affiliations to ground and anchor us as the world around us swirls, shifts, and evolves.

The frameworks I use for understanding how I'm constructed came from fifty years of intensive training with my Councils. They also emerged from my experiences over forty years of having a channeling and energy healing practice, trying to help people find their inner truth and know their unique nature. And, of course, I've learned from lots of teaching and trial and error along the way. Please do not think this means I know the truth. I invite you to play with the information, frameworks, and techniques I am offering here (and in my other books) and see if they serve you.

When we are dead, we can sit around and laugh about what we got right and wrong. For now, I'm not promoting some woo-woo belief system for you to buy in to. I'm just offering frameworks that helped me illuminate my understanding and got me thinking beyond the limits our society has baked into its not-always-tasty cakes.

That said, I believe we each have a Wiser Self. And I believe my Wiser Self belongs to inner groups of teachers (seven groups in my case), which I call my Councils.

To me, Council energy feels collective. Even when a single guide appears to me, I feel the collective energy they belong to and serve. It is not neutral energy either, not just some vague all-wise source. Each Council has a larger purpose or focus to its nature: teaching, healing, framing, connecting worlds, bringing energies into our dimension, keeping history unfolding, and so forth.

Over my forty years of practice, each time I'd channel for someone, I'd tune in to their Councils and speak for them. So I've met thousands of Councils (with many repeats from person to person, of course). And their energy was always vast, but it had clear purpose: to feed our dimension of living from a wellspring of wisdom, knowledge, and energy.

Most people seem to have between one and seven Councils that their Wiser Self belongs to. It doesn't make someone more spiritual to belong to seven or less spiritual to belong to one. These Councils act as guides, teachers, and inner family. I've come to believe that each soul lives multiple lives in multiple times and places, exploring the themes of their inner nature. Many of my fellow Council members are soulmates who I've lived and interacted with in body through these lifetimes, as well as being connected in spirit.

Whether or not this model resonates for you, here are a few important questions to ask yourself:

◆ How can I find what makes me feel alive and seems core to who I am— my nature or my "soul feeds"? (Those qualities tend to represent the kinds of Councils your Wiser Self belongs to. I also call these my "spirit feeds," because they are the specific energetic flavors that nourish me.)

◆ How can I build a life that allows me to express and explore these energies that are core to my nature?

Some of my essences are wordsmith, messenger, teacher/educator, connector, traveler, storyteller, framer, and visionary.

What are your essences? Bridge builder? Peacemaker? Trickster? Lovebug? Starter? Finisher? Details in the middle? Team player? Questioner? Enactor? Archivist? Walker between the worlds? Stargazer?

There are as many Councils—as many essential energetic truths that power our lives and minds and choices—as there are metaphors and understandings of energy, maybe lots more. Anything you do in life, professional or private, small scale or large, that allows you to use your core energies will feed your soul, animate an inner sense of truth, and enrich your life.

Try the guided visit on page 38 to see if it gives you better access to know your Councils. There are two exercises mentioned at the end of this visit, which are useful if you have any reaction to the guided visit. I will briefly introduce them here. You will also find them useful in later chapters when I teach you how to track and balance your story.

Exercise: Clear Fear, Ease Ego, Welcome Wiser Self

This exercise is designed to help you open up to hearing your intuition or guidance. It balances your ego in relation to perceiving energies. It uses a technique I call a "Divine Hook-Up," where you "plug" your left (receiving) index finger into the heart of the Divine (however you picture that, perhaps by pointing upward and outward) and then use your right hand or index finger to bring Radiance, or Source energy, to any place on your body by touching it with your palm or index finger. This creates a circuit to bring Radiance where you need it.

Clear Fear

To clear fear, plug your left index finger into Divine Source (the heart of the Divine or the heart of Mother Earth, for example), and plug your right index finger into the "gamut point" on the back of your left hand. The gamut point sits between the fourth and fifth fingers in the slight indent just below the knuckle (see Figure 1.1). Hold this Divine Hook-Up for a few minutes until you feel a shift and/or release.

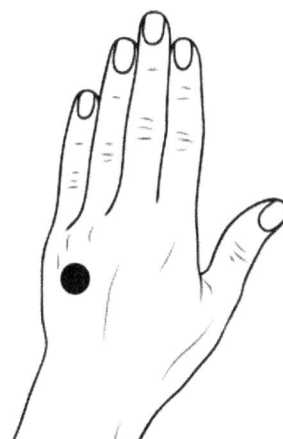

Figure 1.1. The Gamut Point

Ease Ego

To ease ego, do a Divine Hook-Up on the heart, placing your right hand flat on the heart, and plugging your left index finger into Divine Source. Hold for a few minutes until you feel the energies settle or you take a deep breath and relax.

Welcome Wiser Self

To welcome your Wiser Self, picture your Wiser Self behind you, perhaps with their hands on your shoulders as support. Just feel their energy bolstering yours. And, if you would like, you can invite your Wiser Self to step forward and meld with you, encompassing your body like a lovely faux-fur coat!

Third Eye–Belly Button Hook-Up

This is a popular Eden Energy Medicine exercise. Using the middle fingers of each hand, place one finger on your belly button, and the other at your third eye, between and just above your eyebrows. Keeping your fingers on your belly button and third eye, pull upward with both hands. Breathe in through your nose and out through your mouth. Hold until you feel something hook up within you, or find yourself taking a deeper breath, or feel yourself letting go.

Guided Visit: Meet Your Council(s)

To get the most out of the guided visits in this book, you can either record the text for yourself, leaving silent spaces to allow yourself to explore as guided, or you can download an MP3 recording I've provided and use that. See page 13 for instructions on how to access the MP3s.

Shut your eyes, get comfortable where you are sitting, and spend a few minutes breathing in . . . and out . . . just watching your breath and feeling it move in and out of your body.

Bring your attention down out of your head, and dwell for a time in the heart. . . .

When it feels comfortable, imagine you are sitting near some water—it might be a pond, ocean, stream, puddle, or some other form of water. Just notice the water.

Sense further into where you find yourself—don't strain. Just investigate what comes to you about where you are sitting. . . .

If your mind starts to strain or struggle in any way, return your attention to your breath for a few moments, noticing it going in and out . . . and in and out.

When you are ready, invite your Councils to stand behind you. Feel their presence; feel their connections to you. (If this is in any way uncomfortable, shift the scene to feel better—you can invite them to approach from the front, through a tunnel, or whatever is most comfortable to you.)

Ask one Council to step forward and make itself known to you. Ask what you can call them. . . . Ask them what their cosmic purpose is. Don't worry if it makes sense or not . . . just receive what is given, and note it.

If you don't get anything, don't worry. Just know you are planting the question and responses will come in time.

Take some time to communicate with your Council. Ask them whatever questions you may wish to ask. Notice if their communication comes in the form of words . . . gestures . . . images . . . or even just a thought popping into your head. Don't try to control the form of it, just notice. . . .

If you want to write their responses, quietly pick up your pen and jot down notes, trying to keep your mind connected to the energy of the Council. (If you are alone, you can also speak into a recorder.)

Ask them what's the best way to get in touch with them in the future.

Ask them what, if anything, they want from you.

When you are ready, thank them for the visit, and return your attention to your breathing. . . .

After a few minutes of breathing, place your hands on your chest, over your heart, and just sit and feel that physical touch for a few more moments. Hook your energies up by putting one middle finger in your belly button and the other at your third eye, between your eyebrows, and, keeping both fingers in place, pull gently upward.

With each breath in and out, bring your consciousness back into your body, your hands on your chest, your body sitting in this room.

When you are ready, open your eyes.

You may want to take a few moments to jot down any aspect of the encounter that sticks in your mind. Don't try to interpret yet; just record. Do not reject any part of the experience, but notice how you are reacting. If there is any aversion rising in you, Clear Fear, Ease Ego, Welcome Wiser Self.

First, Clear Fear. Plug your right index finger on your "fear point," which sits on the back of your left hand, in the space between your fourth and fifth finger bones. Plug your left index finger into the heart of the Divine, however you envision that. Hold that hook-up until you feel Radiance coming in to calm any fear.

Then, Ease Ego. Plug your left index finger into the heart of the Divine, and place your right hand over your heart chakra, in the center of your chest. Hold that hook-up until you feel your ego release any discomfort.

Finally, Welcome Wiser Self. Invite your Wiser Self to stand behind you, with hands supportive on your shoulders. If you wish, you can invite Wiser Self to step forward and meld with you. Feel the union between your everyday self and your Wiser Self.

• • •

Guidance comes when we let go of the idea that we need some grandiose being to swoop in and give us right answers. Guidance is plentiful when we listen and learn, letting the Universe (or at least our Wiser Self) show us using a rich vocabulary of images, words, music, feelings, direct knowing—fully using the instruments of our body and mind to communicate. Guidance is way more than predictions and right answers: Over time, it helps us shape our knowing, frame our experiences, and develop greater discernment.

When we give ourselves space not to know yet, gathering insights, focusing on one drawstring bag at a time, we can open up to what the inner worlds have to offer us and, in turn, enrich what we can offer to the world around us.

CHAPTER TWO

What's Your Story?

Some years ago, when I lived in British Columbia, a sign was posted in every medical consulting room saying, "One issue per appointment only. If you have a second issue, please make a second appointment." I always shook my head in amazement: How can they hope to heal people if they only know a small piece of what is going on, who we are, what we are living, eating, and experiencing?

Even when I was younger, I was like Great Aunt Myrtle. If you asked me how I was, I wanted to tell you the *story* of how I was, not just summarize how I was with words like "fine," "feverish," or "I have a rash." Why? Because I knew even then that our stories frame and influence what we are living. The elements of character, setting, plot, narrative thread (what connects the pieces), voice, and meaning/purpose all impact one another. When you say goodbye and walk out the door, are you leaving forever or just running out to the grocery store? The same action and words can mean very different things depending on the dynamics of what is unfolding.

A wonderful writing teacher once defined *story* for me. She said, "Take some basic sentences: The girl drops her book. The man comes into the room. These are just experiences. But if you put them in order: The man comes into the room; the girl drops her book—there's a story starting to form. We ask, 'What's going on? Why did she drop her book? Who are these characters to each other?' We feel the energy dynamic forming . . . because of how things got combined."

This notion of story-as-energy-dynamics is key to understanding how to heal ourselves and our world. When we combine words in a sentence and sentences into paragraphs, the elements influence one another and can mean something. Similarly, your body's subtle energies, the energies you are made of, are the building blocks of meaning. When they get put into relationship, into order, into context, woven together, and helped to move the way they are designed to move, your body becomes a web of meaning, a dynamic of stories you are living.

When my Councils introduced the term "story" early in my training with them, it carried this specialized significance. It referred to *how we create meaning by making connections, combining elements, setting a context, and framing our experience.*

When they asked me, "What's your story?" they weren't asking for all the details and data of my experience. They weren't asking me for my feelings about a situation. They wanted me to look at the shape I was giving to my understanding of something—the framework, the dynamics, the motivation, the perspective. What *story* was I living, and how did it affect my evolving self and my day-to-day ability to thrive?

Since our bodies live our stories, then why would the stories *not* have a role in our healing process?

As ridiculous as that administrative decision in British Columbia was to limit patients to one issue per visit, it was not unique. Most medical doctors around the world are constrained by time and economics, even if they want to practice differently. They are trained and funded to elicit medical symptoms and treat the identified conditions, not to listen for the energy dynamics within your story.

And that social norm of treatment removes your illness from the context that creates it. It turns something that is very subjective for you into an objective problem with solutions that may make sense for the symptom but not necessarily for you as a whole person. Our social expectations of illness and healing via Western medicine (as a vast belief system) condition us not to take our own stories seriously—not to even try to hear our bodies communicating and our life expressing what is going on for us.

Hilary came for an energy medicine consultation because she had been diagnosed with heart arrythmia and her doctor had recommended surgical intervention. She was clear she didn't want to have surgery or to take the medication he had offered as a second choice. After she summarized her symptoms and what the doctor had said, I asked, "Tell me about yourself. Tell me about your life."

At first, she didn't understand what I was asking. She wasn't used to having the time and space to tell her story. But, after a few tries, she began to talk about what was going on in her world, in her life, in her mind, and in her emotions. It came out, as she talked, that she was feeling very distant from her husband. And she'd had a big fight with her best friend recently that was making it hard for her to get to sleep at night. She had also lost interest in her work, though it was work she'd historically loved. In general, she had lost the plot of her life. She just wasn't feeling engaged with living, and she was exhausted.

This story gave us lots of other symptoms to understand and respond to in addition to the heart arrythmia. It gave us context for the arrythmia, and it also gave us keys to what was going on for her energetically and how we could use energy to help her heal.

Within Hilary's story, what I heard was the energy of *disconnection.* She wasn't connecting with her husband, her best friend, or her work.

I heard her being *ungrounded.* She wasn't getting nourished or fed by her life. Her work no longer felt sustaining to her.

I heard that she had *lost coherence.* She said, "I can't hold it together. None of this makes sense to me anymore."

I saw that she was experiencing *reactivity.* She had a big fight with her best friend. She was mad at her heart for finking out on her. She was mad at the doctor for offering her bad choices.

But she was also *shut down.* She was saying, "Life is no fun anymore. What does it matter?" She was feeling defeated and didn't have energy to fight the lassitude.

She was feeling exhausted and uninspired. Her well was dry; it was not feeding or fueling her. She was *under-sourced.*

All these issues emerged from her story, in addition to the fact that her heart had literally and symbolically stopped *keeping her rhythm*; it wasn't keeping her *circulation flowing in a balanced way.*

These were all energy themes embedded in her story, not just emotional issues. They showed us the dynamics of what was going on for her in body, mind, and spirit. And it took only a few weeks of doing energy work that addressed these dynamics for Hilary to re-establish a healthy heart rhythm and for the arrythmia to disappear. She did energy exercises that supported *connection, grounding, calming her Gatekeeper, refilling her well, helping her circulation to flow,* and strengthening her Storymaker in general.

Hilary also explored how she could cultivate connection, grounding, calm, inspiration, and better storylines in her day-to-day life. And when those energies were working again, not only was her heart healed, but she was also able to re-engage with the important people around her and find new ways to move forward in her life. Her mojo came back.

Hilary used several exercises to calm reactivity, ground her energy, bring connection, re-establish coherence, and help her heart reset its rhythm. If you are experiencing a need for one of these, try this simple exercise.

Exercise: Coming Home

It is most comfortable to do this exercise sitting or lying down. You can also do it standing, if you are able to stand with your ankles crossed.

1. Place one palm flat on your solar plexus.

2. Leaving your first hand on the solar plexus, place your other palm on your heart chakra (next to your physical heart in the center of your chest).

3. Cross your ankles, one over the other. (To decide which ankle is in front, tune in to how it feels; if you can't tell, it is okay to cross them one way for a time, and then recross them the other way.)

4. Now breathe in through your nose on a slow count of three, and exhale through your mouth on a slow count of five. This is called "3-5 breathing." It can also be done as 4-6 or other counts, as long as you are exhaling longer than you inhaled. Continue this breathing and hold for at least ten breaths.

Tune in to how this makes you feel. You can do this periodically through-out your day to bring yourself home, ground into your center, calm your scattered energies, and reset your rhythm. This exercise also helps bring you back to the present and helps your Storymaker (and your mind) re-establish their priorities.

ENERGY CONVERSATIONS

I go back and forth between calling activities like Coming Home an exercise or an energy conversation. Each energy exercise you will learn in my books, and from other energy medicine modalities you have studied, is, in fact, an energy conversation. I find it helpful to delve into just what is being communicated, to be a bit more conscious of the ways in which I am participating in the energy exchanges that are part of my mind-body-spirit creation of self. It helps me avoid the problem of doing two hours of rote wellness exercises just to cover all my bases!

Let me show you what you are communicating with each step of the exercise Coming Home.

Holding Solar Plexus

The solar plexus is the location of your third chakra, which feeds your creation of self in the world. When you hold it, depending on the intention you are trying to communicate via this hold, you might be calming your expression of self in the world, reinforcing your courage to have a self, containing your energies so they are less scattered, or just showing up in support. Your hand intuitively communicates what is needed. But it is useful to tune in and notice what is being said by both your hand and by that energy center.

Holding Heart Chakra

The heart chakra deals with connection, both your ability to connect with yourself and with others. Think of love as creating strands of connection that flow in and out via this energy center. Holding this center can be consoling, calming, and self-affirming, and holding it together with the solar plexus can help you strengthen the interplay between your heart and the world.

Crossing Your Ankles

Crossing your ankles activates crossover patterns in your energies—which supports your Storymaker, whose job it is to weave energies into patterns. Crossing ankles (or legs or arms or fingers laced together) also helps integrate left and right brain and your active and receptive energies. Donna Eden, an energy medicine teacher extraordinaire who sees energies as clearly as most people see objects around them, has said frequently that the more crossovers you have in your energies, the healthier you are. Hilary's energies had gone "homolateral," meaning they weren't crossing over as needed to keep her story going.

When your ankles are crossed, you are also connecting energy flows (meridians) on the front and inner side of your ankles that feed the liver, kidney, spleen, and pancreas organs and support the issues of *fulfilling your life purpose* (liver meridian), *vitality* (kidney meridian), and *nourishing yourself* (spleen meridian). You are also tying in energy flows on the outside back of your ankles that support your bladder organ as well as the issues of *energy distribution* and *calming your nervous system.*

3-5 breathing

Breathing in through your nose on a count of three, then out through your mouth on a count of five, calms reactivity and interrupts a rhythm that is too fast and galloping away with you. In particular, it calms the vagus nerve, which wanders from brain to gut, influencing the health of everything on its pathway. The reactivity calmed by the vagus nerve generally relates to protecting your inner "sanctity of self"—your sense of safety and security.

Put these all together, and by doing this simple exercise, you are having a profound conversation with your energies.

* * *

Western medicine focused on Hilary's heart but left the energy dynamics and life story issues Hilary was experiencing unaddressed. The myth that our illness or problems reside primarily in the physical symptoms means that often the treatments are limited, despite claims that our medical systems are the best in the world. I have seen lots of people successfully get through serious illnesses using allopathic treatments—cancer, thyroid failure, systemic pain, a replaced joint—only to have some other serious ailment pop up a few years later when the unhealed energy dynamics caused relapses or new illnesses.

It is not the fault of the patient. Our shared Western understanding of illness and wellness has excluded the very things that underlie our physicality: The energies we are made of. The context we live in. The stories we are experiencing. The meaning we are striving to embody. The purpose our unique spirit is seeking to explore.

Most of us also believe that if we have some terrible medical problem going on, we can't figure it out or address it ourselves; we don't have tools to resolve it. I'm not saying here to ignore Western medicine. Sometimes it is very helpful. But if I don't recognize the *myth* that my healing should be in other hands, not my own, I am at the mercy of a very expensive, sometimes very broken system to deal with something as basic and everyday as doing a better job of cultivating and caring for my own well-being!

Energy medicine doesn't ignore the heart rhythms or physical symptoms or diagnoses; it offers us ways to dialogue with our energies, recognize the energy themes embedded within our stories, and support those dynamics to work better.

Hilary's heart arrythmia was not the *cause* of her problem. The arrythmia was the *result* of her energies not moving and circulating and functioning the way they are designed to function. And her symptoms were all typical of someone whose Storymaker isn't working very well or isn't serving them. That was the real root of Hilary's problem. As she learned to strengthen her Storymaker, she was able to heal her heart in all the ways it was ailing. Her body got stronger, and her life was enriched as well.

HOW CAN YOU RECOGNIZE ENERGY DYNAMICS?

Many of us are schooled or encouraged by popular culture to think in terms of feelings and psychological themes, so it is a bit of a shift to think in terms of energy. Here are a few tips to help you learn to recognize energy dynamics.

1. Tell the story.

We are taught in our culture to summarize: Here's what happened and what it means. And we gloss over the dynamics that created the happening and meaning. That flattens our experience to a kind of takeaway: "I went to see my mother the other day, but it wasn't a successful visit." Even in the privacy of our own minds, we tend to rob ourselves of a chance to learn and evolve when we create these generic summaries.

The best way to recognize energy dynamics is to start by telling the story of what is going on. You can write your story, tell it to an exploration partner, or use a voice recorder (on smartphones, there is usually a feature to save the recording as a text file). This is not about creating a masterpiece. Your description may involve just a stream-of-consciousness listing of all the things that seem to be up for you right now, physically and emotionally, in the plot of your life. Or it can also be the kind of tale you put together to tell a friend you haven't seen for a month or two, when they ask, "What's going on for you?" Don't edit your telling. It's fine to add in commentary, including any details that seem random or disconnected.

It is also fine to include both bad news and good, all the contents of what you are experiencing as your "life" right now. You are aiming for subjectivity here, not objectivity: You are telling your story as it comes to you.

Consider what comes out of a real telling of the story. Gillian asked for channeled guidance about how to deal with her mom:

I need some help with procrastination. I have been putting off visiting my mother for a few months; I just couldn't get myself to call and set up a date. So after feeling guilty the whole time, I finally just decided to drop in and surprise her. When I got there, she seemed distracted. I guess she was glad to see me, but you could tell she was just sitting there thinking, "What do you want?"

She kept looking out the window. I found myself staring at my hands and forced myself to look at her and act normal. Inside, I felt like I was going to jump out of my skin. It struck me that she looked a bit like a ghost. Gray. Not very substantial. It was so awkward. I really didn't know what to talk about. And she wasn't much help. She just sat there waiting for me to do all the work.

I got really mad, because here I'd managed to get myself over there, and she didn't seem to care all that much. I left after about twenty minutes, and I think we were BOTH relieved the visit was over.

2. Mine the story for energy themes.

Once you are done writing out your story, take it bit by bit, and ask yourself if there is an energy theme being expressed. (You can also start with overall energetic perceptions if that works better for you.) If you are working with a friend, this is a great exploration to do in tandem, with someone else looking from outside in, while you explore your story's energetics based on how you experienced them.

Take each item in your diatribe or list or story. And ask:

1. Is there a pattern to the energy (i.e., scattered, dispersed, coming in, going out, starting and stopping, faltering, leaking, building up too much pressure, etc.)?

2. What isn't happening that needs to?

3. What is happening that shouldn't be?

4. What myth or belief or storyline is dominating this plot?

5. Does a myth/belief need to be busted?

If you find it difficult to recognize what each piece of the story signals about underlying dynamics, you can underline each key phrase, and then examine it to see what it adds to your understanding of what is going on energetically. Using Gillian's example:

I need some help with <u>procrastination</u>. *I have been* <u>putting off visiting</u> *my* <u>mother</u> *for a few months; I just* <u>couldn't get myself to call</u> *and* <u>set up a date</u>. *So after* <u>feeling guilty</u> *for the whole time, I finally just* <u>decided to drop in</u> *and* <u>surprise her</u>. *When I got there,* <u>she seemed distracted</u>. <u>I guess she was glad to see me,</u> *but* <u>you could tell she was</u> *[just sitting there]* <u>thinking, "What do you want?"</u> *She kept* <u>looking out the window</u>. *I found myself* <u>staring at my hands</u> *and* <u>forced myself to look at her</u> *and* <u>act normal.</u> *Inside, I felt like I was* <u>going to jump out of my skin</u>. *It struck me that* <u>she looked a bit like a ghost.</u> <u>Gray.</u> <u>Not very substantial</u>. *It was so* <u>awkward</u>. *I really* <u>didn't know what to talk about</u>. *And* <u>she wasn't much help</u>. <u>She just sat there waiting for me to do all the work</u>. <u>I got really mad,</u> *because here* <u>I'd managed to get myself over there</u>, *and* <u>she didn't seem to care</u> *all that much. I left after about twenty minutes, and I think we were* <u>BOTH relieved that the visit was done</u>.

Then, if you extract those underlined phrases and sort them, you can often see the energy themes emerging more clearly:

<u>procrastination</u> . . . <u>putting off visiting</u> <u>mother</u> . . . <u>couldn't get myself to call/set up a date</u> . . . <u>feeling guilty</u>	*Lack of clear positive motivation*
<u>decided to drop in</u> . . . <u>surprise her</u>	*Set up a situation with no clear framework*
<u>she seemed distracted</u> . . . <u>looking out the window</u> . . . <u>staring at my hands</u>	*Both lacked focus*
<u>I guess she was glad to see me</u> . . . <u>you could tell she was thinking, "What do you want"?</u>	*Projecting her fears and history onto the visit*
<u>staring at my hands</u> . . . <u>forced myself to look at her / act normal</u> . . . <u>going to jump out of my skin</u> . . . <u>awkward</u> . . . <u>didn't know what to talk about</u>	*Reactivity*
<u>she looked a bit like a ghost</u> . . . . <u>Gray</u> . . . <u>Not very substantial</u>	*Seeing her mom as "not substantial"*
<u>she wasn't much help</u> . . . <u>She just sat there waiting for me to do all the work</u> . . . <u>I got really mad</u> . . . <u>I'd managed to get myself over there</u> . . . <u>she didn't seem to care</u>	*Guilt turned to anger, resentment*
<u>BOTH relieved that the visit was done</u>	*It was not very satisfactory*

In their discussion, Gillian's Councils helped her think about these energy themes within her story:

◆ *Lack of clear motivation.* When we have no carrot or inner motivation pulling us forward, we use the "stick" of guilt to push ourselves to do something.

◆ *You set up a situation with no clear framework.* Rather than coming up with a framework, such as planning a visit where you'd ask her to tell you more about her life, or look at pictures together, you just dropped in, leaving both of you unprepared and unclear how to act.

◆ *Both of you lacked focus.* She seemed distracted; you felt awkward and didn't know what to talk about. While you can't force your mother to focus, how can you support yourself with clearer intention?

◆ *You projected old beliefs (templates) on the situation.* You weren't sure if your mom was glad to see you. You imagined she was feeling impatient, asking herself what you wanted. Is it possible your mother would have acted differently if the visit weren't a surprise, or if you asked her some questions about what she was thinking and feeling?

◆ *Reactivity.* You kept staring at your hands, felt ready to jump out of your skin, got mad, then relieved. Those are signs that your Gatekeeper was trying to protect you.

◆ *Seeing your mom as "not substantial."* What does substantial mean to you? In what ways were each of you substantial in the situation? How much was projection of a ghost, a template of your mother, and how able were you to take her in, in that moment?

◆ *Guilt turned to anger/resentment.* In essence, you were saying, "I pushed past my resistance to you, why didn't you respond and CARE?" Was there a way you could have set up your visit to elicit better caring from her?

◆ *It was not very satisfactory.* Was it possible that how you framed and experienced the situation was influenced by your own resistance to being there, so it couldn't really satisfy any deeper sense of yearning or purpose in you?

3. Address these energy themes with energy work and lifestyle adjustments.

We talked it over to find some energy work that could help Gillian heal this story. Although this situation revealed Gillian's feelings about her mom, the *disconnect, lack of framework,* and *lack of motivation* that she called "procrastination" was, in fact, a pattern. It showed up in other parts of her life and in her physical health in the form of skin problems (*container/framework* issues), recurring bouts of brain fog (*focus, disconnect*), and difficulty recovering from viruses (*reactivity/Gatekeeper imbalance, lack of motivation to move forward*).

The energy work she chose included working on *finding more positive motivation in her life,* trying to make choices based on the carrot not the stick—asking herself several times a day, "What do you want to experience?"

She practiced *how to make a framework* that allows both her and her mom to contribute. Instead of a spur-of-the-moment drop-in, she decided to plan a visit focused on asking her mom to talk more about her own experiences growing up.

She spent about five minutes each day doing some symbolic figure-eighting (see page 8) between her and her mom to *create better harmony.* She also used a photo of her and her mom sitting together and doodled "frames" around the two figures, encasing them in shapes like squares, figure eights, and circles to signal to her brain the connection between them.

It was so obvious from her story that Gillian needed to *clear out outdated templates* about her mom from the past. They were interfering with her ability to even see her mom in the present. We set up an appointment to use energy medicine to track and balance this story in a subsequent visit (see chapter 8).

Gillian set a goal for herself of *learning to stay present* for what is, connecting to a present circumstance. Once she recognized what she was projecting onto this situation from her past, she decided to take a few moments throughout the day to stop and ask herself, "What story am I living now? Who are the characters, and what roles am I assigning to each of them?" She'd also ask herself, "How have I framed what is or isn't happening? How does that serve me or cause me grief?" Then she'd ask, "What story do I choose to live in this moment?"

After this long discussion, her guides asked Gillian to now retell the story. Here's what she came up with:

I always wanted a mom who was warm and fuzzy, and enthused about me. When I was a kid, my mom filled her life with volunteer activities, and there were six of us, so I always felt invisible. Now that I'm older and see my sisters with their kids, I wonder if she wasn't just overwhelmed most of the time. Once I left home, I didn't look back for a long while. There were many years when I didn't even have contact with my mom. I told myself she didn't care, but I have to admit, she sent me occasional notes and cards—more than I did for her. I'd always get mad about the cards because they seemed so impersonal. But if I'm being honest, that's not entirely fair: My mom was respecting the rules of engagement I set up myself.

So although I called it procrastination, you're right. I was not clear on why I was visiting. I wanted to be the kind of person who visits. But I was still mad at my mom for all the ways I felt ignored. And so I guess it makes sense that I would go visit but also "ghost" her or, at least, turn her into a ghost. I can't tell you much about the actual woman I visited. I was so uncomfortable. She seemed so OLD, and frail, and disengaged from everything, not just from me. It scared me, so I just detached from the situation and told myself it was the same old same old. I guess I should add "detaching" to my list of energy homework and explore what it means to feel attached!

A BRIEF GUIDE TO RECOGNIZING ENERGY DYNAMICS

It is something of an art form to recognize energy themes and dynamics. For some people, it is intuitive and easy; others may need to practice how to think on this level. Energy themes generally describe how energy is working and/or what purpose it serves.

Often your language, particularly idioms, will show you what is going on energetically—for example, "I can't hold it together" (*lack of coherence*), "I am at the end of my rope" (*low on resources*), and "I am over the moon" (*expanded energy, filled with Radiance*).

It is useful to try to come up with a metaphor to describe how you feel or how your energy is behaving—for example, "I feel like I've been run over by a ten-ton truck" (*lack of space for energies to move; collapsed energies*), "I'm a fish out of water" (*unsourced, inadequate container*), or "I feel like an engine that's been taken apart, and they forgot how to put it back together" (*lack of connection, integration*).

Here is a brief guide on what to look for. Energy dynamics often relate to these functions, each of which I'll describe in more detail below:

- Sourcing
- Movement
- Connection
- Containment

- Protection
- Framing
- Integration
- Change

Sourcing

Are you/your energies being fed, nourished, and sourced, or are they in deprivation? Are you able to metabolize what feeds you and release what does not?

Quick exercise: Do Clear Fear, Ease Ego, Welcome Wiser Self on page 37. By plugging your index finger into the heart of the Divine and bringing that energy to various parts of you, you are juicing your Radiance, or Source energy. And, by inviting your Wiser Self to meld with you like a big faux-fur coat, you are submersing your body in energies that are true to your nature.

Movement

Is the situation/body function moving or stuck, circulating, short-circuiting, flowing, moving in some kind of patterns, blocked, dispersed, or failing to move? How is it moving, and is that appropriate for your body, mind, and spirit?

Quick exercise: Do a Touch Bath, touching and tapping your body all over (like a sponge bath only using energy). Then, with your flat palms, do a Body Sweep:

1. Trace up the front of your body from your toes to your collarbone.

2. Trace from the front of each shoulder out the soft, inner side of your arm and hand to your fingertips.

3. Trace with your palm along the backs of each arm, from fingertips to backs of shoulders.

4. Starting at your forehead, trace up over the back of your head and down your back to your heels, then sweep the energy off your baby toes.*

You can finish by figure-eighting (see page 8) every which way in your aura, the energy field that surrounds your body like a protective space suit.

Connection

What is connected or disconnected, collaborating or working against each other, sporadically connecting or connecting in an unhealthy way, coherent or incoherent, grounded or ungrounded, or anchored or lacking moorings?

Quick exercise: Try "Healing Hands":

1. Rub your hands together, and ask one hand, "Where do you want to go?" Let the intelligence in your hand guide where you place it on your body (or field).

2. Then ask your other hand, "Where do you want to go?" Again, use the wisdom of your hand to guide placement.

3. Hold those two spots for a while, just tuning in to the communications and what you are feeling.

4. Then ask each hand, in turn, "Do you want to move, or stay where you are?" Shift your hands to where they want to go, letting them create the pattern of holds and connection.

5. Keep this up until you feel a sense of completion (or run out of time).

---

* Thanks to Stephanie Eldringhoff for this Body Sweep exercise.

Containment

Is the energy/dynamic contained or unbounded, leaking out or seeping in, or too strong for the container or not strong enough to power the ship? Is it adequately and reasonably filtered? Are you open or closed?

Quick exercise: Create a "Smart Filter" along the edge of your aura.

1. At arm's length from your body, figure-eight toward and away from you to reinforce the filter that sits at the edge of your aura.

2. If you wish, add a color to strengthen the quality you want to put into your smart filter.

3. If it's too much work to figure-eight the whole large area, call on helpers—elves, fairies, UPS delivery people, and the like—to help complete the figure-eight protection and containment of your aura.

Protection

Is there any reactivity protecting you from outer threats and guarding your inner sanctity? Is there adequate communication, safety, identity, and/or distribution to allow you to create meaning?

Quick exercise: Trace hearts on your heart chakra area, then do 3-5 breathing (see page 46, #4) to cultivate a sense of safety.

Framing

What is the belief, intention, interpretation, or myth that is motivating you and others in the story? What are the terms of engagement?

Quick exercise: Listen to whatever you are telling yourself about the situation. Is it a belief that allows you to change, expand, shift, evolve, and/or thrive? If not, reframe the statement to allow for more spacious possibility. You can use something like "Even though I am feeling like nothing ever works out for me, every experience of success and failure serves as grist for my evolving soul."

If this is too "thinky," you can also use your hands to trace shapes that feel sacred to you around your whole body: diamonds, hearts, circles, spirals, squares . . . whatever feels like a shape you crave to frame your experience.

Integration

Are the parts woven, frayed, integrated, collaborating, or working at cross-purposes?

Quick exercise: Do Celtic weaving around your whole body and around a symbolic representation of your life.

A Celtic weave is basically a dual figure eight, with both hands weaving in, crossing each other, and then weaving out in unison (see page 93). You can also sing a scale up and then down multiple times. This tells your energy systems to organize and helps them collaborate.

Change

Have the old norms broken apart or been amended? Are new habits or influences needing assimilation or disrupting your rhythms? Do you recognize where the energies are in the cycles of inception, expansion, expression, and return, or other cycles of nature?

Quick exercise: Try Shifting Cycles:

1. In the air in front of you, slowly trace a large clockwise circle, representing winter at the bottom (six o'clock), spring on the left side (nine o'clock), summer at the top (twelve o'clock), and autumn on the right side (three o'clock). See Figure 2.1. Start with whatever season you intuitively feel is your best starting point. (Don't worry, you can't do this wrong!)

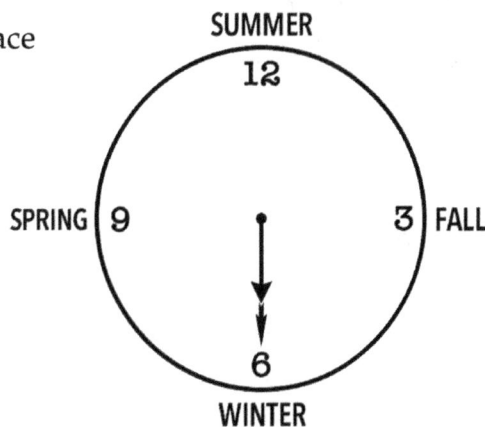

Figure 2.1. The Seasonal Clock

2. As you draw the circle, if you encounter places where the tracing feels sticky or impeded, stop and figure-eight that sticky place.

3. Then, imagine the situation you are trying to change is sitting inside that circle. Figure-eight between you and the situation you are picturing.

4. Then continue drawing the circle slowly until you have traced the whole circle through all the seasons.

5. Repeat this until you can trace the full circle without feeling any hitches.

|||||||||||| **Play with It!** ||||||||||||

It is often easier to see energy dynamics for someone else than it is for yourself. When your cousin is going on and on at a family dinner, you are probably thinking something like, *He needs a good filter,* or *His on-off switch is broken.* These are both ways of characterizing what you are picking up about his energy, apart from the content of what he's putting out.

Play with this story about my recent adventures. See if you can perceive any energy themes or dynamics. Was I having issues with sourcing, movement, connection, containment, protection, framing, integration, and/or change? Remember, energy is a language, so you can also use your own vocabulary to characterize any energy dynamics you perceive within the story—you don't have to stick to that list!

You also do not need to find *all* the dynamics—if you just recognize one, that would be enough for you to help me get started dialoguing with my energies and supporting them.

Last week was a week of things going wrong for me! First of all, my toilet wasn't flushing all the way. I was so tired of having to hold the handle down, I finally called the plumber to come fix it. He poked around and discovered the water pressure on the house was sky high—over 100 when it should be 60 to 70. He said, "Your pressure valve that moderates water pressure on your house has failed." Geez, ka-ching! I asked him to replace the valve *because it had to be done, and then he replaced the toilet, which had gotten blown out. Then he snaked out a bunch of clogged drains. And $6,000 later, my toilet flushed.*

Then I was driving home from the store and a message came up on my screen that my tire pressure was off. I contacted a guy to rotate my tires, and he discovered the pressure was dangerously low—24 instead of 42. But at least it turned out the tires didn't need rotating. That was good.

Then I lost two days of work because I just felt like I was going to explode with tension. I couldn't relax. Something was off, but I couldn't figure it out. And my eyes were hurting like crazy. I had serious eyestrain.

I went to the eye doctor, who diagnosed me with glaucoma. He explained that the eyeball pressure gets too high because with age (I'm in my sixties), the surface of the eye becomes less permeable. He explained that it is incurable (his belief system, not mine) and my choices for treatment were eye drops I might or might not tolerate, eye drops that would turn my eyes yellow, or laser surgery that would punch tiny holes in the surface of my eyes and need to be redone every three years or so. . . .

I feel like my eyes and ears are both shutting down lately. Maybe it's because the news is so toxic, and I keep tuning in to it. My hearing seems to be failing. My eyes are tired. I just don't want to let the world in right now! I indulged in a few hours of panic and then looked up my notes on energy medicine for eyes.

Remember, there are no right answers. But if you regularly ask yourself, "What is going on for that person energetically?" you will come to see the energy dynamics underlying the "data" of the story. Remember, tone of voice, body language, context, and your larger knowledge of a person can also come into the equation to help you recognize what is happening with their energies.

Here are some themes I came up with:

◆ In my story, I hear the energy of *discontinuity*. I kept getting stopped by things going wrong and being off-balance, things needing to be addressed.

- I hear the theme of *tension being off.* My tires, eyes, and emotions are all too tense or not tense enough.

- I hear the theme of *pressure.* My tires were too low, house pressure too high, my eyeballs were too tight, life felt stressful.

- I hear the theme of *broken "permeability"—the in and out, release/taking in was not working right.* The toilet was only half-flushing. I felt a need to shut out the world because it was overwhelming me. But when you shut stuff out, you also shut yourself off from what needs to come in.

- I hear the theme of *details going wrong because of larger issues* (framing). The broken toilet was, in fact, a whole-house valve issue. The glaucoma was due to my tissues overall getting less permeable (according to the ophthalmologist). His frame did not fit my belief system about what is healable.

- I also heard a theme of *strain—things only half-working, not being fully on.* My toilet could flush, but only by holding the handle down. My eyes and ears and tires worked, but it was a strain . . . I was straining to hear and straining to see with my tired eyes.

- And another theme was *needing to call for help, maybe "need for better maintenance."* I called a plumber, saw an eye doctor, and got the tires checked.

These are not the only possible themes. You may have come up with something else entirely.

What are some simple energy "conversations" I could have with my body-mind to address these energy dynamics? What would you do if you were experiencing strain or discontinuity, and so forth? Here's what I did:

- To address *discontinuity*, I traced large and small figure eights all over my body and in my energy field. Figure eights speak to your energy systems, inviting even flow, continuity, and integration. I could have used circles, spirals, or other shapes that expressed *continuity* for me.

- To address *tension*, I did a kind of self-massage, spreading my skin apart in various directions wherever I felt tight. It was a gesture of opening up and creating space (and permeability).

- I used 3-5 breathing (see page 46, #4) to calm the *strain* and to slow down, so I wasn't straining to get my work done.

- And I did the exercise Celtic Clearing (see page 105) to release garbage that was *clogging* my works. I also addressed the pipes and tires on their own terms, which helped release my sense of being clogged physically.

- For my eyes, I addressed the broken *permeability* by cupping them with my palms many times a day, warming and moistening the tissue, listening to them, and letting them show me what else they needed to help them heal.

Since eyes are the window to the soul, this diagnosis gives me rich territory to explore over time. How can I better balance the interplay between my soul and the world? I can feel the muscles of my face, including those around my eyeballs, are *too tight*. I can tap and pulse energy all over my face and around my eyes to invite those muscles to release and relax.

● ● ●

You will be learning many more energy conversations and tools to address energy dynamics. For now, feel free to experiment with how to respond as you identify energy themes and dynamics in yourself. Usually just having awareness of what is happening energetically is a good first step toward transforming the situation. If you notice *energetic fatigue*, for example, then you can find many creative ways to bring in antidotes: rest, inspiration, change of scenery, new pace, enlisting helpers, new terms of engagement, and the like.

Energy dynamics often respond to symbolic energy communications: Make up a gesture or style of touch or bring in a color to see if that shifts your energies and changes the dynamics you have noticed. Play with your entire vocabulary of movement, gesture, touch, image, sound, symbol, and more to address an energy issue you are exploring.

Healing your story is not about fixing what's wrong with you or even correcting energies that aren't working. It's about entering into the conversation as the creative artist you are and evolving the ways your energies can move and interact to form a richer, more satisfactory body-mind-spirit experience.

CHAPTER THREE

Creation

The same year Josefina took me to meet the Tibetans, a friend invited me to accompany her to an ashram in Oakland to meet Gurumayi, the new "girl guru" many of my friends were swooning over. I'd never been to an ashram before, and this one was a good introduction: friendly, well organized, colorful, and large. I'm guessing there were more than 500 people there. My friend explained that Gurumayi would lead us all in meditation, and then afterward, people would line up and we could each have a moment of one-on-one with the girl guru, possibly to receive *shaktipat*, a kind of transmission of spiritual energy.

I was curious to see what this was all about—not the religious aspects of it, but what her energy felt like. My own training had been so focused on my Councils that I wanted to know how this teacher-in-body operated. We gathered quietly to sit on cushions on the floor in the main hall, beautifully decorated with flowers, with incense wafting and quiet Hindu music playing. It was clear most of the people around me were regulars; they were already focusing inward, preparing for the meditation. A few "tourists" like me, I noticed, were gazing around them, some apprehensive, some looking giddy or hopeful. I settled in to pay attention to my breath, as I'd learned from my meditation retreats.

After about ten minutes, a peaceful looking Indian man, wearing a kurta pajama, came to the front and announced, "Gurumayi cannot join us today. We will meditate for half an hour and then play you a video of her."

Oh well, I thought. *At least it's a nice space for meditation.* But almost as soon as I settled into my cushion, I felt this weird tugging at my shoulder blades and in the small of my back. I twitched them slowly, pretending I was just stretching my back a bit, but the tug continued. I surreptitiously turned my head to see if someone was behind me, trying to get my attention for some reason. But all I saw was a row of meditating yogis.

Then, out of the corner of my eye, I saw Gurumayi (her spirit at least). She was up near the ceiling, kind of sitting and floating. And there were bands of light streaming from her hands, connecting up to each person in the hall, at the small of their back and their wing bones. She was weaving her hands in and out, which created a huge weave in the strands of light, connecting everyone there in a gorgeous rainbow web of light. I thought, chuckling to myself, *Well, I guess you showed up after all!* And to my embarrassment, she looked right at me. I said to her (in my mind): "How do you do that?" She smiled kindly, and said, "Why don't you just let yourself feel this and be part of it? There is no obligation. Just a chance to be in this moment with the others."

Right. I shut my eyes and returned my attention to my breathing. And I felt a deep calm and peace. I felt myself woven into the beautiful fabric, together with the 500 people, mostly strangers, who were sitting together and trusting this practice. I remember thinking, *Cool! I'd like to learn how to do that!*

What Gurumayi was doing that day, albeit in spirit, was weaving together the Storymakers of each person there into a collective awareness. She was creating a unified field of energies out of our disparate selves, giving us, for that moment, a sense of profound community and belonging, a deeper awareness of being in the right place at the right time. The video they played afterward explained that the purpose of her teaching was not to make us fall in love with her. Instead, by activating our feelings of love, her goal was to serve as a mirror, to wake us up to our own beauty, our own energies, our own potential.

I didn't ever return to the ashram (I was not particularly attracted to the rituals or guru worship), so I never got to meet the girl guru in person, but I felt deeply grateful for that lesson in awakening—and for the demonstration of how important the "Web of Connections" is to our individual sense of orientation and well-being.

This story came back to mind vividly last year. I was at a conference and attended a keynote presentation offered by a man whose promotional materials call him a visionary, a leading light of next level energy medicine. I was curious about what he had to say and wanted to learn more about his work. He claimed, as several other thought leaders have been claiming lately, to have cracked the codes of energy healing. For some reason, code-breaking is a popular guiding metaphor these days, as if energy were a deeply encrypted language. But I believe that it is more accessible than that. It is our mother tongue and the basis of how we navigate our reality moment by moment.

At any rate, I once again found myself in a large hall, awaiting the arrival of a person heralded as a kind of guru. This time, there were about 300 people present, and the folding chairs were more accommodating to my comfort-loving body. A glowing, extroverted, super-enthusiastic announcer came onto the stage to introduce our speaker, reciting his impressive bio with high praise, and then pounding music began to play, so loud, I could feel the beat of it pulsing through me. People around me were perking up, getting excited. I could see an adrenaline glow forming around the room. It reminded me of those large high-roller-style marketing seminars, whipping up enthusiasm with music and hype.

And then the speaker came bounding out as if parting the waters, looking humble and grateful for our recognition of his status as a vaunted dignitary. He was perfectly coifed, glowing with good health—a model of what he was promising us: high energy and high performance.

As he spoke, his voice was like a snake charmer's flute, alternating between wonder at the amazing experiences he'd had to open his awareness and confidence in his science-based authority. Although it was clearly a set speech with PowerPoint slides for each point he was making, he kept insisting that he was channeling, that this sharing he was doing was a transmission, a download, *just* for us, and that we were being initiated into understandings it had taken him *years* to learn. His speech got faster and faster, more and more insistent, like the pounding music he'd entered on. So fast, there was no time to stop, to ask, "Does this make sense?" No time to compare what he was saying to what we already knew or thought. It was a masterful delivery.

I was curious. Was he perhaps showing me another way to weave or animate people's consciousness? Around me, the crowd was clearly excited. I heard someone behind me say, "This is worth the price of the whole conference!" But I didn't see any Web of Connections; I didn't see a weave at all. In fact, what I saw was a room full of excited people pulsing with adrenaline but slightly detached from their core. And many people's energetic steering mechanism, their Assemblage Point, was skewed. Slightly off-center. This mechanism (see page 192) is our guiding light, a North Star. If it is off-center and you steer toward it, you can end up wildly off course.

I tried to keep an open mind. I really did. There are many ways to understand and present energy healing. His message was almost opposite to how I've come to see energies. He explained, with lots of pictures from ancient cultures mixed with pop-quantum science, how we are formed from the outside in. Our energies come to us, he explained, from "out there" in the cosmos and work their way in toward our centers. He claimed that this vision came to him from his guides, though I must confess I'd heard two other speakers make the same claim that month, and that he was sharing it to help us "uplevel" our consciousness even as we sat there that evening. (His language, not mine.) And many of my colleagues were moved, feeling awe and gratitude, so it is possible I just wasn't ready to uplevel.

My perception has always been that our energy emanates outward from our core. Because of how I've experienced guidance, I see even energies from *out there* as coming through me *in there*. Not that energies don't also reach us from out there. It's just not how I see us constructed.

And that's my point, again: The story we use to frame our reality, our creation, greatly influences how our energies work and what choices we make. Each of these gurus was setting the terms of engagement. What I observed in the first instance was a teacher whose methods were giving her students a chance to experience community and deep peace. In the second instance, I saw a teacher whipping his students to a frenzy but energetically skewing their steering mechanisms, leaving them less capable of perceiving truth or evaluating the information they were getting.

I should mention, the issue wasn't just excitement versus calm. If the second speaker had been a Sufi teacher, leading us in whirling dance, perhaps the frenzy would have healed and supported our Storymakers, our ability to connect, to steer our ship, and that would have been a different story.

At any rate, in this era when we are seeing a proliferation of self-appointed gurus claiming to be able to give us the keys to happiness, wellness, success, and cracking the codes of our very existence, we still need to be able to hold our own in the face of energies coming at us. We need to be able to set our own terms of engagement and care for the instruments of body, mind, and spirit that allow us to come into form and experience life in its many dimensions.

I have written elsewhere that I believe we are collectively in a transition from a world rooted in outside-in thinking to a world where we live more comfortably from the inside out. We are needing to learn both how to discern when outside authority is reliable and also how to find our inner authority (authorship) and wisdom. Maybe that's why the girl guru's approach was more appealing to me than the motivational speaker. It was a more inside-out approach.

TRINITY: STORYMAKER, GATEKEEPER, AND RADIANCE

My Councils refer to this inside-out view of us when they say we humans are *creators*. We are constantly creating our lives, assigning meaning and mining experience to learn from it. We are dynamic, evolving, multi-dimensional beings, enjoying some time in this earth dimension.

It is not my intention to try to convince you this is more correct or a better model than other frameworks. Certainly, I don't think it is some kind of cracked code. Instead, I just want to show you how the simple framework my Councils have taught me allows us to work with our own energies and to help our world heal.

In a way, it is a kind of non-denominational creation story. It starts from our center. At root, we have consciousness. Consciousness is the life force, soul juice, the Radiance that animates us. It is the ghost we give up when we "give up the ghost."

To have this body-based, earth-based experience, our consciousness has two main mechanisms that I introduced earlier:

1. The Storymaker, which creates and codifies the frames and stories (energy dynamics) we are living

2. The Gatekeeper, which protects and preserves our body-mind-spirit instrument and the stories we are creating

All three parts of this trinity—Radiance, Storymaker, and Gatekeeper—are constantly learning, adapting to circumstances, and co-creating your life and your world with others. Your consciousness (Radiance) uses your Storymaker to weave your body's energies into coherence so you have physical health and well-being. It also uses your Storymaker to weave your mind into meaningful stories that frame your life and identity. It is this evolving creation that your Gatekeeper protects and maintains.

GATEKEEPER

If you think of your Gatekeeper as being similar to the immune system—as your physical, emotional, energetic, and spiritual immune system, protecting and preserving the artwork that is you—you can probably see what I mean when I say it is a multi-dimensional mechanism. That's because we are familiar with the immune system and are used to hearing about its intricacies.

Your Gatekeeper keeps the gates of self. It says: *This can come in; this must stay out. This is safe; this is a threat. This is part of my identity; this is an invader.* Gatekeeper has four main tasks:

1. **Protection:** It keeps you safe.

2. **Maintaining your identity:** "This is me, this is not me."

3. **Maintaining habits:** It is part of your autopilot.

4. **Distributing energies:** This is done according to the patterns established by your Storymaker.

Like the immune system, Gatekeeper can affect all your body-mind functions: digestion, circulation, fight-flight-freeze-and-fog reactivity, nervous system, thinking, perceptions, and feelings. In energy terms, it can affect or be triggered by an imbalance in any of your energy systems, such as your aura, meridians, and chakras. Your Gatekeeper can disrupt your energies and will also react to energetic disruptions.

Here are three short exercises that help calm your Gatekeeper and reset reactivity:

Exercise: Consolation, Version 1

1. Place your right hand on your left side, with your little finger at the base of your rib cage and the rest of your hand above it.

2. Place your left hand flat along the left side of your face, cradling that whole side of your face, with the heel of your hand at your jawline, your thumb curled behind your ear, and the rest of your fingers extending upward in front of the ear, covering your temple. (See Figure 3.1.) Hold until you feel consoled, or you feel something settle within you.

3. Repeat this hold in reverse, holding your right rib and the right side of your face. Experiment with how each feels.

Variation: If it is too difficult for you to reach your left rib with your right hand, you can use your left hand on the rib, and reach across to cradle your face with your right hand, little finger curling behind your ear.

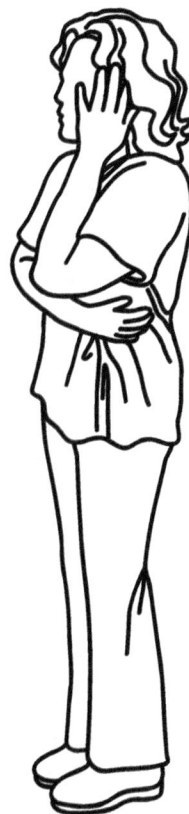

Figure 3.1.
Consolation, Version 1

This exercise has long been one of my go-to exercises when I am lying in bed, trying to let go of the day and get to sleep. It calms your Gatekeeper via your rib cage, which acts as a container for your heart and lungs and spleen and liver (organs that work 24/7 on your behalf), and also anchors it into your Storymaker via the side of your face, one of the anchors you will learn about in chapter 4.

Exercise: Expanding Hearts

1. Imagine you are trying to calm your dog or cat. Begin by petting yourself slowly and lovingly up around and behind your ears and down the sides of your neck. This calms your body self (your "earth elemental self"). Breathe slowly, and maybe croon to yourself (if you have the privacy), "good girl" or "good boy."

2. Now, bring your hands over your heart, holding both your physiological heart to the left of center and your heart chakra in the center. This is a Storymaker anchor but also a center for your "yin Gatekeeper," the part that protects your inner sanctity of self. (Yang Gatekeeper protects you in the world). Connect into this anchor, let your hands speak to it, and listen in to the dialogue between your heart and hands.

3. Then, very slowly, start tracing hearts there on your body with whatever pressure feels loving and supportive. As you do this, you can rock back and forth slowly to help calm your Gatekeeper further and set a peaceful rhythm for your heart and mind. (This is especially helpful if your blood is racing and your adrenaline or cortisol levels are up.)

4. After a few minutes of slow heart tracing and rocking, slowly and gradually expand the size of each heart to include more area of your chest, torso, neck, and upper legs, and finally to encompass your entire body. You can continue to expand to trace hearts on your *home*, *life*, and *world* too.

5. End by bringing your hands back to your heart, and just sit there, breathing in a 3-5 rhythm (see page 46, #4), and feeling the space you have created with your hearts.

This exercise speaks to your earth elemental self (your physical, creature self) and addresses both your yang Gatekeeper, protecting you from invaders, and your yin Gatekeeper, protecting your inner sanctity. Stroking behind your ear and doing the 3-5 breathing and rocking help to calm your vagus nerve and your Gatekeeper in general; the hearts activate your Storymaker to address the energy dynamics that triggered you.

Tip: Note that this exercise, like most of the energy medicine tools in this book, is not just for calming emotional reactivity. If you find yourself getting congested, itchy, or having other immune system reactions, this can help calm your body as well as your mind and spirit.

Exercise: Porcupine Reset

If you have followed my work elsewhere, you will be familiar with this exercise. I teach it in most of my classes and books as a great way to quickly reset your Gatekeeper. I am including it here because you will be using it as you learn to track and balance stories later in this book. You can view a video of this exercise at ellenmeredith.com/storyline. Password: cominghome.

When you get triggered into fight-or-flight reactivity, the energies in your aura flip polarities. It is like in the show *Star Trek*, when the spaceship *Enterprise* is being attacked by Klingons. All the power is funneled into the shields to protect the ship. In the case of your body, your energies turn outward for protection, rather than orienting inward to fuel the workings of your ship, your body. And, in this state, you look like a porcupine. Porcupine Reset takes you off red alert and brings the energies back from the shields to once again serve your body's functioning. Here are the simple instructions. See corresponding Figure 3.2 on the next page.

1. Starting at the top of the head, grab the energy with two hands. [1]

2. On the inhale, pull it straight up to arm's length. [2]

3. On the exhale, pull it down on either side of your body, arcing out in an egg-shaped arc. [3]

4. Tack the energy to the floor. [4]

5. Grab energy from the earth. [5]

6. On the inhale, pull up with both hands, arcing out. [6]

7. On the exhale, tack it to the top. [7]

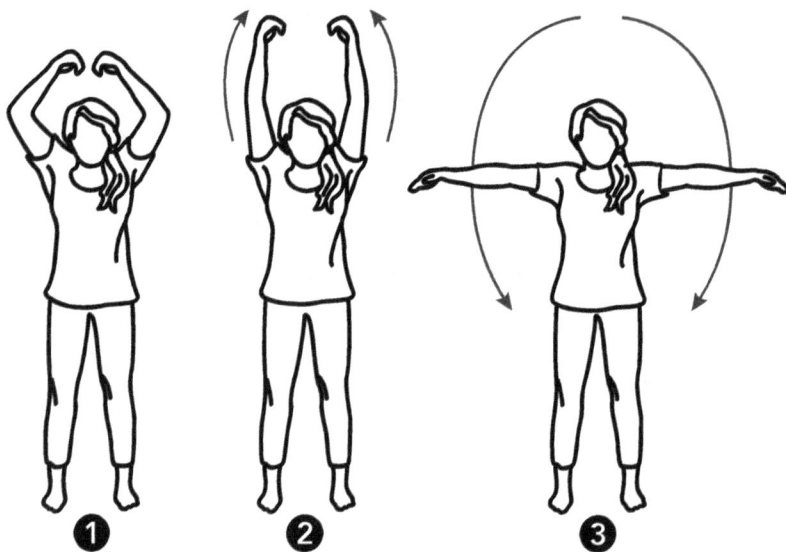

(1) Starting at the top of the head, grab the energy with two hands.

(2) On the inhale, pull it straight up to arm's length.

(3) On the exhale, pull it down on either side of your body, arcing out in an egg-shaped arc.

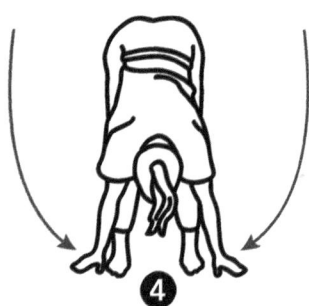

(4) Tack the energy to the floor.

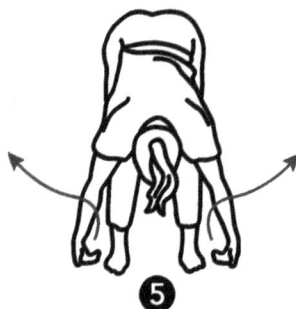

(5) Grab energy from the earth.

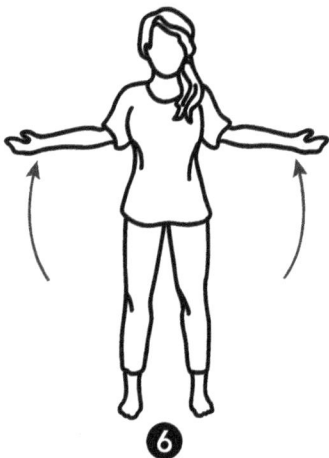

(6) On the inhale, pull up with both hands, arcing out.

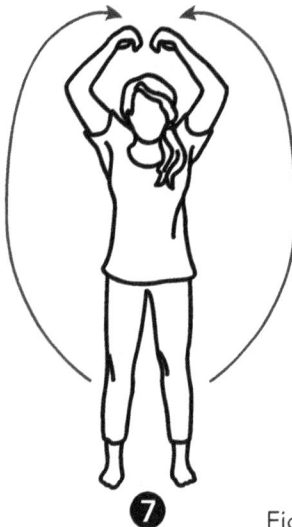

(7) On the exhale, tack it to the top.

Figure 3.2. Porcupine Reset

THE STORYMAKER

You will be learning many more tools in this book to work with your Gatekeeper and to bring it into better collaboration with your Storymaker. However, the main character I want to focus on at the moment is your Storymaker, the part of us that we're less familiar with in our culture.

The Storymaker is your mechanism for setting the terms of engagement—it enables you to create and shape an identity and a life. It is your mechanism for putting together the stories your body lives. It has six main tasks:

1. **Anchoring:** keeping body, mind, and soul together.

2. **Framing:** setting the terms of engagement, including creating your mental, emotional, and physical identity and life; includes setting up patterns and habits.

3. **Weaving:** connecting elements together to construct meaning; creating webs of connection and meaning, both within you and between you and others.

4. **Sourcing:** bringing in/selecting the resources that will support you.

5. **Steering:** creating and navigating your storyline(s) and steering the body and mind in physical and mental space.

6. **Learning:** distilling meaning from experience and creating templates of experience together with your Gatekeeper to run your autopilot.

When your Storymaker and Gatekeeper operate as they should, it is a marvel. When these mechanisms are dysregulated, skewed, blocked, or broken, life becomes less tenable. Stories are not just narratives in our brain. They are energy dynamics we live, within every fiber of our being, throughout our many dimensions of self. So it becomes imperative to learn about the vast and very cool equipment you have to work with your story on many dimensions. That's where we're heading.

What a Dysregulated or Broken Storymaker Feels Like

Most of us could serve as poster children for a dysregulated or broken Storymaker at some time or other. Who doesn't need to occasionally adjust our anchors and grounding? Who doesn't need to revamp the frameworks and beliefs that guide our thinking and choices, the integration of energies and weave that keeps us feeling whole and renewed? Most of us need to adjust our ability to feel fed and connected to resources, the path we are steering. And most of us have to upgrade how we learn from our experiences.

Almost every ill we suffer in body and/or mind and in our social exchanges has elements of Storymaker dysfunction and Gatekeeper reactivity. That's why I think it's useful to address the Storymaker in ways that strengthen it generally while also working with the specialized tools for supporting healthier anchoring, framing, weaving, sourcing, steering, and learning.

Here are just a few stories to start us off:

Mel's Story

Mel grew up in a small town, where as far as he knew he was the only gay man. He knew from an early age that he was different, and he was one of those truly androgenous kids who just couldn't hide how different he was. He was bullied, taunted, and sometimes physically hurt by a certain group of boys, who, unfortunately, were in pretty much every one of his classes throughout their school years. Fortunately, Mel's parents sent him away to a summer camp for gifted children each summer, where he discovered other kids who were different, unusual, and not always comfortable in their skins. There he experienced wonderful bonding and a sense of community, only to return home each August to the misery of his small-minded school and town.

At the age of sixteen, Mel left home after applying for early admission to college, and once again, he was blessed to find like-minded others as well as support for his sexuality and style of expression. He studied social work and psychology and became an advocate for kids living on the streets, especially young LGBTQ kids who had experienced the same kinds of pain. His friends knew him as a nuanced, sophisticated, funny, loving guy, dedicated to helping others, and considered him an important person to have on their team.

But Mel suffered from periodic bouts of depression and exhaustion, as if someone had pulled the plug. Sometimes he could stand up to opposition, and it made him stronger and more determined. But if a comment, look, or interaction with someone who was bullying and gaslighting people hit him wrong, he would come apart at the seams. He'd be that hurt, lost kid again. He'd hide out at home, trying to talk himself off the cliff.

Mel had created a new self that was extremely high functioning and positive in the world. But he also had some brokenness and special vulnerability in his anchors and core weaves. They showed up periodically and wreaked havoc in his ability to inhabit the self he had created.

Belinda's Story

Belinda was diagnosed with lupus when she was thirty-two years old. This came up after she had four relationships break up in five years. Each time, she could see that although her own behavior was not blameless, she had chosen someone who was not available to her for various reasons: One partner was a compulsive over-worker, another was still in love with a previous girlfriend, and a third was just self-absorbed and only responded well when Belinda gave up her own needs and wishes to please him. The fourth was controlling and put her down to make himself feel powerful. Each time she started to date someone new, her friends tried to warn her about what was going on. But Belinda's ability to recognize the terms of engagement were dysregulated, and she carried a framing belief that she wasn't worthy of love.

In addition, Belinda's steering mechanism was chronically out of balance. She continued to make the same mistakes over and over, because she kept using incorrect maps and wonky equipment to steer her ship. The lupus forced her to stop dating and to seek help to get her Gatekeeper rebalanced. Auto-immune illness is both a Storymaker and Gatekeeper issue.

Both Melinda and Mel had Storymaker vulnerabilities that caused their Gatekeeper to stop funding forward motion in their life. Mel's Storymaker had a gap between his childhood experiences and the newer identity he had created. He was inadequately anchored. His reactivity took the form of depression and energetic shutdown. Although he could usually talk himself back into his newer comfortable identity, he lived in fear of falling back into the nightmarish reality he'd grown up with.

Belinda's Storymaker wasn't strong enough to sustain her due to damage to her framing mechanism that affected her sense of self-worth. Her Gatekeeper went into overdrive, attacking her own cells and making her ache all over and begin to lose her hair—which did not help her self-esteem after so many breakups.

There are as many symptoms of Storymaker dysregulation or breakdown as there are stories to tell. And most involve a one-two punch: Storymaker can't do its job, so Gatekeeper goes into *protect* mode and spoils the party.

Here are some typical ways you might feel if your Storymaker is not functioning well. I'll be diving more fully into each task of the Storymaker in coming chapters, so you'll get more familiar with recognizing what is going on behind the symptoms.

If your Storymaker isn't working correctly, you might feel like you are coming apart at the seams, dissolving, disintegrating, disconnected, or lacking coherence.

You might wake up to the fact that you've been operating under an illusion, projecting a false story onto a situation to make it conform with your own chosen frameworks. You might not wake up to this fact, but instead find it out from friends or when you don't get that promotion you were expecting.

Your nervous system might make you feel constantly jumped up or its opposite, deflated and hopeless. And you might see addictions come into play where you are reaching for a substance or behavior to self-medicate.

You might find yourself getting fixated on details, losing track of the plot-line, falling down a rabbit hole, and unable to move comfortably between the bigger picture and the small details. You might similarly find yourself unable to handle details because you are fixating on some goal or larger vision you don't know how to reach.

Any time you act out of character, lose track of where you are in time and space, go through a significant shift in your literal or figurative voice, lose a sense of continuity, get mired in other people's opinions, find yourself tied up in knots, unable to see things from both other people's point of view and your own, find yourself yearning for shortcuts (wanting someone else to fix you), or not remembering how to enjoy the journey, that's a clue your Storymaker is off-kilter.

When you can't distinguish your own story from someone else's or project your storyline onto others, not knowing your own truth, or find yourself having slippery ethics, not being able to tell right from wrong, or trying to manipulate others (e.g., codependent, controlling, passive aggressive), your Storymaker could use some help.

If you can't feel your successes or experience an overblown impact when you fail or get negative feedback, you chronically lose hope, or you have a need for other people's approval over an intrinsic sense of satisfaction from having an experience, your Storymaker is out of whack.

If you find yourself more comfortable with virtual reality than lived experience or find yourself addicted to screens, gossip, or political wrangling, rather than craving time spent using your senses and inhabiting your body, your Storymaker has lost the plot.

In this era of massive change, we have an epidemic of disconnection and of dysregulated Storymakers. It means that:

1. Many people can't discern lies from truth and are easily manipulated.

2. We can't form coherent positive narratives that make sense for our own soul's purpose and that support planetary well-being.

3. We get triggered and flip into survival mode (our Gatekeepers are running rampant, and we are vulnerable to viruses, other people's programming, and chronic illness).

4. The weaves that hold us together are coming loose or insufficient.

5. We get dysregulated in our brains: as evidenced by brain fog, nervous disorders, obsessive or compulsive thinking, pace dysregulation

(speeding up, slowing down, arrythmia), addictive behaviors, and lack of proportion.

6. Weak links in our body start to express the stress: joints (arthritis), muscle problems, headaches, injuries, and so forth.

When what we try to create gets picked apart, denied, gaslighted, decontextualized, attacked, polemicized, and manipulated with AI, as is happening a lot in this time of change, and when we hear over and over how the world is going to hell in a handbasket, it creates a form of repetitive stress injury to our Storymakers.

Fortunately, there are wonderful, creative ways you can start, in this moment, to support your Storymaker to thrive and steer your ship.

Exercise: Consolation, Version 2

1. Reach across your body with your right hand and place it on your left side, with your little finger at the base of your rib cage and the rest of your hand above it. (See the tip on page 81 if this is uncomfortable for you.)

2. With your left hand, hold hands with the Divine, however you picture that. You can literally hold on to something (e.g., the paw of a stuffed animal or a corner of your pillow) or just do the gesture while imagining yourself hand in hand with the Divine. If you are an atheist, hold hands with what you hold sacred, such as nature, truth, or kindness.

3. Now, imagine you have vertical boxes along each shoulder blade (on your wing bones). Shake your shoulder blades a few times to open those boxes, and unfurl your angel wings that are tucked in and stored there. You can flap them slowly back and forth to help your wings spread out.

4. Then, gently, wrap each wing around yourself, like a loving blanket. Swaddle yourself in the magic of your angel wings, feeling them around you like a cocoon, holding you.

This exercise helps give you a sense of sourcing, framing, weave, and anchoring in particular, but it is just a great way to give support to your Storymaker by connecting it to the Radiance of Divine consciousness.

Tip: If you have difficulty reaching these areas of your anatomy, you can ask a friend or practitioner to hold your left rib cage, together with your scapula. While they do this hold, you can hold hands with the Divine. Connecting these two parts of your anatomy helps strengthen your physical container (the rib cage) and connect it to your potential (your wing bones). Holding hands with the Divine helps bring Divine guidance into the conversation. Repeat this exercise on both sides of the body.

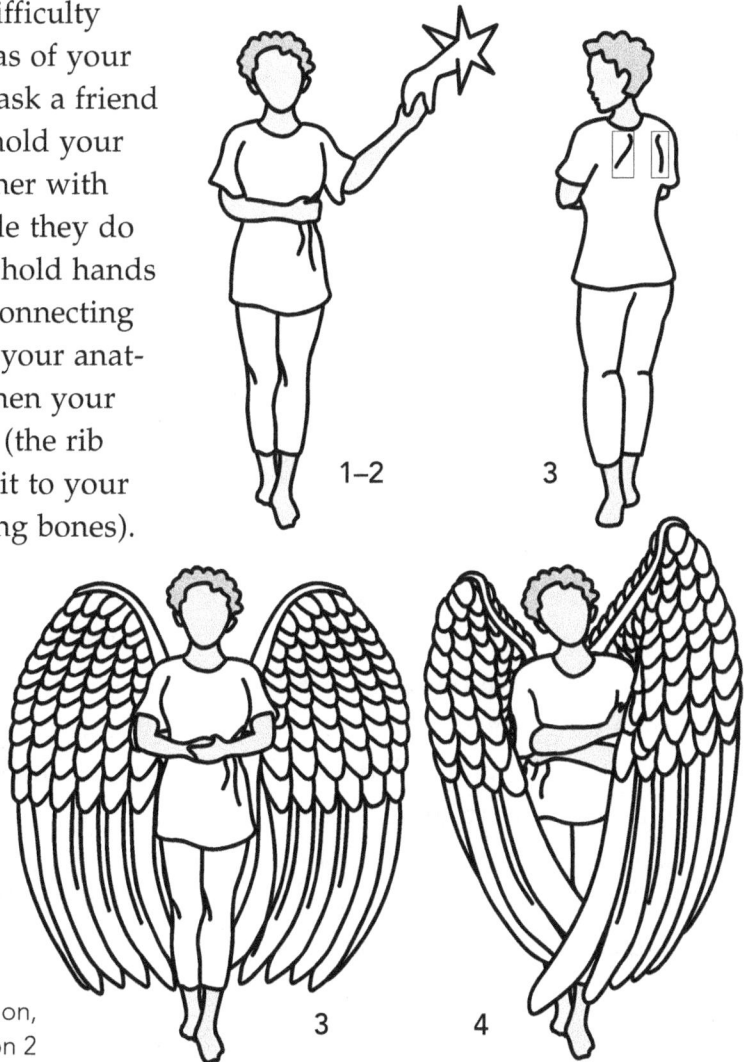

Figure. 3.3. Consolation, Version 2

Like the exercise Coming Home on page 46, both versions of Consolation help you anchor your mind into your body, and anchor your spirit into your body and mind.

MULTI-DIMENSIONAL HEALING

My Councils regularly remind me, "You are part of us, and we are part of you." They mean by this that "I" live on many dimensions, and at the dimensions where they live, I am (my Wiser Self is) part of their collective consciousness. The same is true for you and your Councils.

Some Councils feel closer to our dimension, and others are more distant. I avoid hierarchical categories when possible, so I call the more distant ones "Council's Councils." Councils are at a good level to be able to give us wisdom, perspective, and guidance, but also to have some idea of what it means to us to be living viscerally and walking each step of the path they are recommending.

If a teacher is too distant from our dimension, a member of a Council's Council, for example, I have found that the guidance may be a bit too abstract or not all that workable in my lived experience. They are less personal, and I have to keep in mind that what they are suggesting, while wise, may take my entire lifetime or several lifetimes to step into and really embody.

I once asked my *Teachers and Travelers* Council (who specialize in cross-fertilization of cultures), "How is it that you speak such good English?" They responded, "We are finding the language in your head." *Duh! Cosmic eyeroll.* "Our own language is closer to metaphors."

"Is it like pictographs?" I asked. They said, "It is more like holograms of consciousness, in multiple dimensions. The closest your mind comes to that is the ability to use and understand metaphor."

This made sense to me; it was an aha moment. When I was in college studying creative writing, I spent an entire semester just writing metaphors—page after page of them. I couldn't craft a poem or story to save my life. But I would wake up in the night with metaphors just pouring out of me. They would often arrive with story fragments—parts of plots, small sketches—in which the metaphor was like a gem, gleaming at me and overshadowing its setting. It was embarrassing to have to turn in such raw material when other students were saying something with poems and stories. But that semester I just had nothing to say, despite pages and pages of ways to say it.

Luckily, my teacher at the time was a poet. He loved metaphors and was fine to just let me capture the flow. He told me the story of a poet he knew who would write metaphors and snippets on little pieces of paper and put them in a box. A couple of times a year, she'd feel a quickening inside her, pull out the box, and spend days just playing with her snippets and crafting poems.

That never happened to me. What happened to me was that a year or two later, I began hearing and dialoguing with my Councils. It was as if their consciousness, their language, preceded them. By awakening the parts of my mind that could intersect with theirs, we were creating a bridge for conversation and for them to begin my training.

The awakening our shared world is going through is, in part, a process of preparing us to understand new perspectives, of breaking free from the linear, patterned thinking that has dominated our shared reality. Many individuals and groups have been trying to find new configurations, new language, and have been getting to know more dimensions of the self. They have developed more understanding of the ways our stories play out on many levels.

It is a group effort. Although there are some downsides to people's multiple escapes from reality, including into video games, superhero tales, fantasy fiction, spiritual woo-woo experiences, role-play, and more, the upside has been a stretching of our ability to take in new ways of understanding what it means to be alive, to be human, even to embrace our superhuman potentials. Like writing metaphors, it is giving our younger generations, in particular, more flexibility of mind and spirit to wake up to their multiple dimensions.

Of course, I should mention a major downside: When you apply the hierarchical, power-over value systems of our crumbling patriarchy to this impulse to create new ways of being, you can get radical violations of people's humanity—terrorists who believe their vision and values trump our shared humanity and give them the right to destroy things. They are willing to use threat and force to impose their own forms of rigid top-down control. This is true in the political realm, of course, but it is equally true in spiritual hierarchies where visionary leaders use methods of delivering their teachings that interfere with their followers' ability to steer their own ship.

What are the many dimensions of self? This concept has been explored in many spiritual traditions and some psychological systems as well. Of course, from Freud we have the theory of id, ego, and superego (not my favorite configuration) as places where healing might need to happen. From the voice dialogue method and similar therapy techniques, we are taught to identify and name various sub-voices within us and create dialogue among them.

Some spiritual systems identify locations of types of consciousness. For example, the layers of the aura that surround your body are often spelled out in specific terms: etheric body, emotional body, mental body, astral body, etheric template body, celestial body, and ketheric/causal body.*

However, I'm a bit leery of these seemingly precise anatomy-of-the-spirit configurations. Since energy is always moving and learning, and is an expression of consciousness, those locations are not fixed, nor is their purpose always the same. And certainly the colors and rate of vibration and those kinds of details differ for each of us. Even physical anatomy isn't fixed: I know a woman whose organs are all reversed from the normal placement in the body. Her heart is on the right side, liver on the left, and so forth.

My Councils always referred to the exploration of dimensions of being as travel in the "Country of the Mind." Of course, they were referring to the larger concept of mind, including everywhere the mind touches and can touch. And so I find it useful to keep an open mind about those realms, identify a few rough landmarks, and see what I discover.

In chapter 8, when we explore how to work with templates of experience, you'll use levels of the chakras as landmarks to find your way through dimensions of your being. Those roughly correspond to locations in time and space of your creation of self: now, recent days, this phase of your life, the story or frames you have placed on your life, the contracts you came in with, your multiple lives (past selves, counterpart selves), and your cosmic dimension. But I think it's best to learn initially through experience and explore the Country of the Mind to see what it has to teach you.

---

* Tanaaz, "The Seven Layers of Your Aura," Forever Conscious, accessed October 18, 2024, https://foreverconscious.com/7-layers-aura.

Being able to travel within the dimensions of yourself allows you to learn from your multi-dimensional self and, where needed, to bring integration and healing.

Tune in to your body and find a place you are drawn to where you can take a sounding. As in the exercise Taking Soundings on page 32, you can place your hand on that area and ask an open-ended question such as "Give me insight into . . ." Or you can just tune in and see what you perceive.

Now, treating your chosen place as a doorway or passageway, travel through it to explore what you find there. If you want to invite your Councils along to act as guides, feel free to do that. Otherwise, just explore at your own pace on a self-guided tour.

Here's an example:

> *I feel drawn to my left kidney/adrenal gland, and I place my hand over them on my back. I take a sounding, and it feels cold and still, closed down or closed in on itself somehow.*
>
> *I look for a doorway and immediately see a small wooden door on the far right-hand side at the back. Opening the door, I step through into what looks like a huge birthday party. There are multicolored streamers hanging from the ceiling. My Councils are there, and also my younger self, my Wiser Self, my inner critic (wearing those plastic Groucho Marx glasses with a fake nose and moustache), and a few of my cats who have died. There's an air of excitement. People are congratulating me, but I'm not sure what for. I'm not sure what is going on. Then they start to hold hands and form into a line, and they wrap themselves around me in a spiral. One of my cats (Cleo) has wrapped herself around my neck. The other (Pudge) has laid down on my feet.*
>
> *My Councils say, "Put your other hand on your solar plexus, and twist counter-clockwise." I do this and feel my pent-up energies releasing, my sense of self expanding.*
>
> *For the interval of about seven deep breaths, I just inhabit that space.*

Then I get curious about what is going on in the right kidney adrenal space, so I thank everyone, enjoy a group hug, and bring my hand and attention to the other side. There, the outer side is also cold and sterile feeling. Too quiet. But when I open the doorway, at the center in the back, what I see is a long corridor, green, green, green, reminding me of a country road in France, lined with trees. I ask my Councils what is down that road. They say, "Your vacation place." I'm not ready to go there yet, so I take a few minutes to breathe in the smells of the trees and grass, feeling the promise of a relaxing vacation, then return my awareness to my hand on my body.

Some people travel easily in the Country of the Mind. If you can, let yourself just explore and experience without expectations or a need to get anything. And if you are one of the people who just draw blanks when you try to explore like this, investigate the quality of the blank, as that may be the part of the Country of the Mind you are being invited to visit. Is it comfortable? Stressful? If you find yourself getting reactive, do the exercise Consolation, Version 1, on page 71 with one hand on the left side of your face and the other on the left side of your rib cage. Sometimes, just locating a door or passage or being willing to try is a significant step.

To end your explorations, do the exercise Coming Home on page 46: Place one hand on your solar plexus, the other hand on your heart, cross your ankles, and do 3-5 breathing, in through your nose and out through your mouth. This is a great way to reconnect with your everyday self.

You might want to take a few minutes to jot down in your journal what you experienced. Generally, the mind takes time to catch up with the experiential self, so allow yourself to experience without needing to categorize or find the significance. Sometimes the meaning will come to you later, maybe even a few days later. Sometimes the importance of the exploration is what it does to your energies to spend time in various outposts of your multi-dimensional self.

Note: This exploration uses doorways in the body, which I find is a good starting point for developing your skills as a traveler. If you find yourself being pulled into other landscapes, doorways, or passages, and are comfortable with that, you can of course explore the Country of the Mind you access that way. Just remember to bring guidance along and to keep an anchor on your body in the form of a hand touching some part of your anatomy. If you are the kind of person who thinks the more far-out, far-flung regions of consciousness are the juiciest, invite yourself to explore what you can discover when you start closer to home.

● ● ●

Shifting from a view of yourself as some kind of machine or system that needs to be repaired to one in which you are creating a self and co-creating a world gives you myriad ways to work from the inside out to heal yourself and the world.

Knowing you have a Gatekeeper and Storymaker, being used by your consciousness to create and maintain your body and mind, gives you new ways to address situations that are both very physical and ones that seem more existential.

In the coming chapters, we will dive into the Storymaker more deeply and look at how working with your anchoring, framing, weaving, sourcing, steering, and learning gives you new ways to heal your body, mind, and spirit. We will also weave in how to bring your Gatekeeper into better alignment with your chosen creation of self.

CHAPTER FOUR

Anchoring

"My husband always thinks he knows what is best for me." She's brandishing a sharp metal pick as she says it, in the midst of cleaning my teeth the old-fashioned way, without lasers. My hygienist, Maria, started the session in her usual professional and contained manner. Then, once we got underway, she cleared her throat a few times and let me know it was probably her last time cleaning my teeth.

She's been having bouts of fatigue, she explains, sometimes so strong she's had to call in sick. And her husband has been insisting it's because of her job and she needs to quit. At first, she says to me, "So I'll probably be turning in my notice soon."

With sharp metal implements scraping away in my mouth, I can't say much. I *mmmph* in a sympathetic tone. And then the story just keeps coming.

"But," she says, "I love my job. He doesn't understand. It has been my identity for so many years, and I feel I can actually do some good here."

She is getting increasingly agitated, and I find myself gripping my chair, willing the pick not to slip. I'm trying to back off subtly from her scraping action to lessen the pressure on my gums.

"And of course, he never considers whether *he's* part of the problem." Her tone starts to sound a lot like the laser I opted to avoid. "I get home, exhausted after a day of work, and somehow, it's still my responsibility to get everything ready for dinner, even though *he* retired six months ago and could be stepping up at this point to do more. Instead, he wants me to give up what I do. And I'm ten years younger than him!"

This is the point at which she brandishes the pick in the air, and I decide to intervene. "This is a super-upsetting situation," I say. "Can I teach you a simple energy exercise that might help?"

Surprisingly, she says yes. So I invite her to hold both knees and just breathe in through her nose and out through her mouth. I ask her to tune in and see what that feels like. She is visibly calmer already. "Good," she says. "I don't know why I was getting so worked up."

I suggest she try holding one knee while placing her other hand on her back, on the area called the Mingmen, behind her belly button. As she does that, I can see her professional self click back into place. She holds the other knee together with her Mingmen, and shakes her head as she does so, saying, "I'm sorry. I don't know what came over me." She's clearly embarrassed.

I invite her to hold both sides of her face. As she does so, I can see the moment when compassion rises, and she forgives her lapse. And she's baaaack.

Who among us hasn't been on both sides of this situation? I have certainly found myself swept away by a story from somewhere else in my life taking over my present reality. In fact, I have to be especially careful that doesn't happen while I drive, which seems to get my mind traveling as well. And most of us have found ourselves in dramas where we are unwitting or unwilling stand-ins for someone who isn't even there—where someone's rush of reactivity spills over on us, sometimes in threatening ways.

Maria's Storymaker was out of balance; it was dysregulated. And because of that, her stories were skewed and her Gatekeeper was triggered into reactivity. You might be asking, "Wasn't it telling the *story* that knocked her off-balance?" Possibly. It can go both ways: If you live through a shocking event, that can leave your Storymaker acting wonky and needing readjustment. Like when you drop a guitar—you generally find it needs to be retuned, if not repaired. But the opposite can also happen. If your Storymaker goes out of tune, then the stories you are living start to reflect that distortion. Like your gait going lopsided when you have a stone in your shoe.

In any case, in our culture, with its emphasis on talk therapy for the mind and medication to quiet symptoms in the body, we mostly default to trying to analyze the story or shoot the messenger. Instead, if you can learn to retune the instrument, start again with clear purpose, focusing on the tone and energetics for a few moments, you can reset your Storymaker, shift the energy dynamics, *and* have more creative options for living your stories.

It is quite magical to see someone like Maria brought back home to herself, back into balance. It's not always so simple—but often it is, especially if you dialogue with your energies regularly: They can respond rather quickly to subtle invitations and supports.

The places I invited Maria to hold are part of a set of Storymaker "anchors" that seat the mind in the body and serve as rich places to meet up with spirit. By holding them, she was able to come home to herself, reconnect her body and mind, and, at least temporarily, retune her Storymaker and free herself from the sway of a story that destabilizes her sense of self.

Was it a permanent fix? Probably not. She would have to use this tool over time to train her Storymaker to stay steady. I see it like brushing my teeth. Brushing them once might clean out the guck from dinner, but it probably won't prevent decay over time. On the other hand, if I brush as needed, at least once a day and in general after meals that stick in my teeth, I'm going to need less help from my dentist!

When my Councils suggested I write this book, the first tool they proposed I include was the protocol Storymaker Reset. The holds I showed Maria are a part of that exercise. Different parts of your body act as doorways, entry points for fruitful dialogue and adjustment. The Storymaker anchors allow you to retune (and strengthen) your Storymaker, like the pegs of a guitar giving you access to tune the strings. The Storymaker Reset protocol is the original pattern of holds they suggested.

Protocol: Storymaker Reset

The anchors of your Storymaker include:

➤ Soles of each foot, particularly the arches

➤ Both knees

➤ The Mingmen area on your back opposite your belly button (between vertebrae L2–L4)

➤ Your heart chakra (next to your anatomical heart in the center of your chest)

➤ The sides of your face

➤ Your "thinking cap"—the top of your head from above your ears to your crown

Storymaker Reset involves a series of holds and energy conversations. You can take your time and really tune in to each hold. Where possible, use your flat hand or palms.

If you can't reach an area, you can use your fingertips or ask a friend to help. For the Mingmen area, you can place a wadded-up sweater or stuffed animal (something with good energy) in that area and sink into it while lying or sitting down.

Preliminary

If you are doing this exercise as first aid, proceed to the numbered steps below. If you start doing the holds and can't feel yourself *clicking in* or making real connection, first try one of two things:

➤ Flip your hand back and forth over the area several times, touching each time with the front and then back of your hand. This resets the polarities of positive and negative charges. Reversing these is a common trick the Gatekeeper uses to shut down access.

➤ If that doesn't give you access, imagine there is a jar lid on the balls of your feet, knees, Mingmen area, and heart chakra. Grasp the lid, inhale, and gently pull the jar lid slightly away from the surface of the anchor area about a quarter inch. Slowly and carefully jiggle the jar lid (also known as a "sonar ring," which I teach about in *Your Body Will Show You the Way*). Then, on your exhale, gently reseat the jar lid on the surface of the anchor. Knocking your sonar rings off-kilter is a more advanced way the Gatekeeper, when in reactivity, can mess with your ability to connect body, mind, and spirit.

Storymaker Holds

While these Storymaker holds can be done standing or lying down, I find it easiest to do these holds while seated on a couch where I can bend my knees and reach my feet. Remove your shoes if possible. Follow the sequence from 1 to 9, holding each area for one to three minutes, or until you feel you have made contact and *arrived*.

1. Hold both knees, hands cupping each kneecap.

2. Hold each knee in turn together with the Mingmen area.

3. Hold the bottoms of your feet with your palms on the arches of each foot. You can hold one at a time if you can't reach both.

4. Hold each foot arch together with each knee: left arch to left knee, left arch to right knee, right arch to right knee, right arch to left knee (you can use your intuition to decide in which order to hold these).

5. Hold the arch of each foot together with the Mingmen area.

6. Hold each foot arch together with your heart chakra.

7. Hold the two sides of your face, cradling it in your hands.

8. Hold the two sides of your head, your thinking cap. Place the base of each palm above each ear, with your fingertips meeting at the top of your head (where the soft spot is on a baby).

9. End with a slow, heartfelt Celtic Weave (see next).

Exercise: Celtic Weave

This is an Eden Energy Medicine exercise that I have modified slightly. A Celtic weave in energy medicine basically involves tracing a dual figure eight, with both hands weaving in, crossing each other, and then weaving out in unison. Imagine you are conducting an orchestra with both arms figure-eighting in toward each other and crossing. Then your hands rotate and you figure-eight outward again.

Note: If you find it hard to coordinate the double eights, start by figure-eighting with one hand, then as you travel inward with that hand, add in a figure eight with your other hand, also traveling inward. The figure eights cross over at the center and create a motion of weaving in and out with both hands.

Reminder: View a video of this motion and exercise at ellenmeredith.com/storyline. Password: cominghome.

In this version of the exercise, you will Celtic-weave four parts of your body: *your face, your torso, your knees,* and *your ankles/feet.*

To start:

1. Stand with your hands on your thighs. Breathe in through your nose and out through your mouth throughout this exercise. Swing your arms around in a big arc and bring your hands into a prayer position.

2. Rub your hands together to activate energy. Bring your hands up facing each side of your head, about six inches away from your ears.

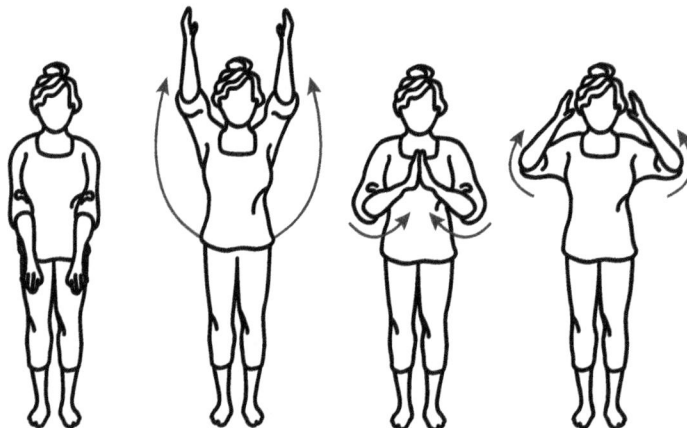

Celtic-weave your head:

3. Inhale deeply and bring your elbows in toward each other and continue with your upper arms crossing in front of you. Exhale while turning your hands and weaving outward in a smooth motion, extending your arms as if embracing the world. This weaving motion is called "Celtic weaving" in Eden Energy Medicine.

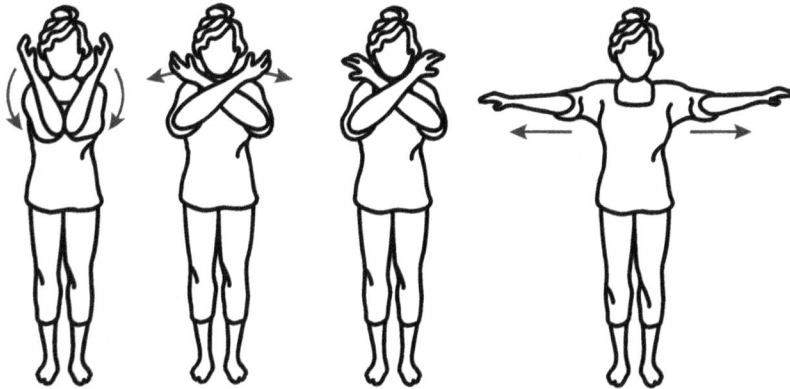

Celtic-weave your torso:

4. Inhale, and Celtic-weave at your waist and lower torso, bringing your hands in to cross in front of you. Then, exhale to weave the energy outward again and extend your arms back behind you like wings.

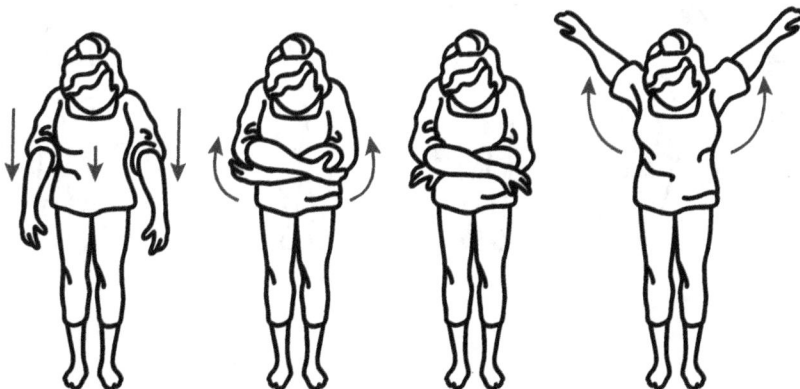

Celtic-weave your knees:

5. Bend down to repeat this Celtic weaving motion at your knees. Inhale and bring each hand inward toward each other and then crossing. Exhale, and weave the energy outward.

Celtic-weave your ankles:

6. Repeat this weaving motion at your ankles. Inhale and bring each hand inward toward each other and then crossing. Exhale, weave the energy outward, this time extending your hands out and back behind you.

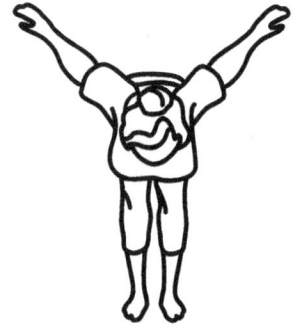

Integrate the weaves:

7. Now, on the next inhale, scoop up fresh Source energy from the earth, and bring it up above your head. With your exhale, let the energy you've scooped up shower down all around you, spreading it with your hands as you weave double figure eights (like in the caduceus) from head to foot.

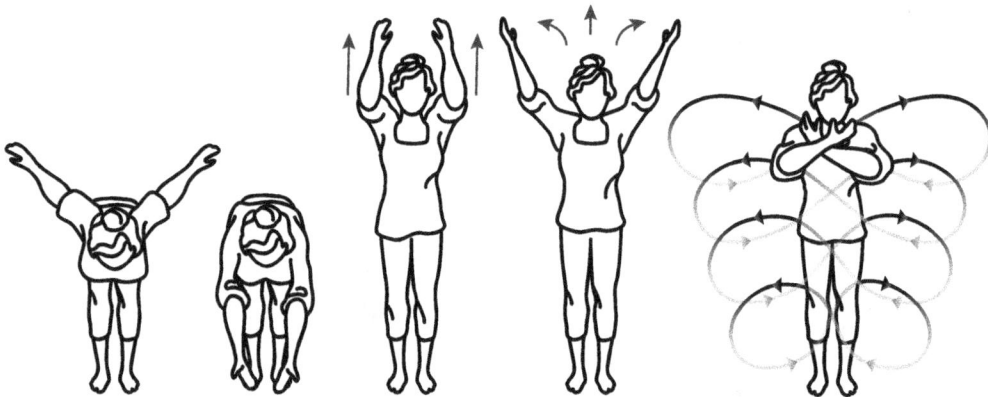

The Storymaker anchors are infinitely flexible, and you can also work them individually or with just a subset, as I showed Maria. This is great for first aid when you are losing the plot or your energy dynamics (your stories) and are spiraling out of control and need a quick way to re-anchor. I frequently just grasp one knee for a time or place both hands on the sides of my face, cradling it, and let that bring me home to myself.

The full pattern of holds just described gives you a way to do a more thorough renovation of your Storymaker, reinforcing your mind-body connections that frequently and easily fall apart. It also anchors spirit more firmly into body and mind. When Mel, the gay activist I talked about in chapter 3, found himself knocked off his foundation because of a gap between who he had been growing up and the self he'd created, he found it helpful to do this full pattern twice a day for a while. It allowed him to reassemble his disconnected Storymaker and bring it into alignment with his chosen values. He was anchoring his chosen identity into this basic mechanism for integrating energies to create meaning. And it was a drug-free way to pull him off the floor and out of depression.

HOLDING BODY, MIND, AND SPIRIT TOGETHER

Remember, *anchoring* is one of the six tasks of your Storymaker. It refers to holding body, mind, and spirit together, to the seating of your mind and spirit into your body. Once anchored, the mind and body can work together, and spirit can make itself heard.

I have other names for this phenomenon of body, mind, and soul holding together: Glue, Honey (as in what holds the layers of baklava together), Communion, Coherence, and Presence. And, like with Maria, presence is what flies out the window for most of us when our Storymaker goes out of tune and our Gatekeeper gets triggered.

With musical instruments, often the finer the instrument, the more easily it goes out of tune. That's true for our human instruments as well. We are easily destabilized because we are made to be fine instruments, flexible and capable of playing the music of our souls in ways that do us justice.

That's where anchoring comes in. It is how we make sure our different dimensions are in sync and working synergistically. My Councils always feel like a collective consciousness to me—not one single guide but a group of spirits. And when you think of it, we are each kind of collective ourselves as well. We've got our body consciousness, anchored in our earth elemental self, or our creature nature. We've got our minds, able to travel in imagination to all kinds of places and dimensions (talking self). And we've got our Wiser Self that inhabits the realm of spirit or soul. And it's a challenge sometimes to get those three parts of us on the same page, working well together.

When you slip out of that alignment, your Gatekeeper sounds the alarm, and you can experience all kinds of symptoms:

- Feeling fuzzy and disoriented
- Allergic reactions
- Feeling itchy or achy
- Coming down with whatever your body uses as a chronic flag
- Migraines
- Gut or stomach issues
- Flare-ups of old injuries
- Depression, lethargy, and fatigue
- Breaking out in rashes
- Feelings of being lost
- Feelings of anger

You may have your own weird but effective flags—any chronic symptoms or behaviors or thought patterns that show up and can't be traced to a single cause because they arise in response to being out of balance or alignment.

As I list these symptoms, I hope you're thinking, *Hmmm, symptoms are really flags, telling me that something is not working correctly in my construction of self.* Probably you weren't thinking that. But it's true. When your gut is spasming or refusing to work, it is not just a gut issue: It is also a flag of energy imbalance.

In our culture, we usually ask, "What triggered this?" But I think we need to add *flags* to our concept of illness. Triggers are generally rooted in cause and effect: You have an allergic reaction—what triggered it? How can you avoid it in the future?

Symptoms are most often the result of your Gatekeeper protecting your creation of self. And these are flags—they may or may not relate to a food, pathogen, or specific trigger. Like the straws on the camel's back, they can signal that you have slipped out of balance and now your Storymaker can't carry the load. Your Gatekeeper flags it using its broad and sometimes ugly vocabulary of signals.

When your skin breaks out, there could be a bug or bacteria triggering that reaction, but whether it's a bug or an imbalance between body-mind and spirit, it is always your Gatekeeper sounding the alarm, saying, "What is me? What is not me? I can't tell!" Even when you are feeling you can't breathe, it's often not a problem with your lungs per se; it is the energies that are supposed to keep your lungs running that are being diverted into protection mode and interfering with your everyday body functions.

What this means is that you can use energy medicine to heal almost anything and find great relief from most illnesses. The task is to support your Storymaker and calm your Gatekeeper by getting your energies moving in healthy patterns and integrated into a whole. When someone asks me, "How can I use energy medicine to heal my [name the disease]," the answer is always the same: We need to support your construction of self. And often that starts with making sure that body, mind, and spirit can communicate and come into shared purpose.

"GAS CAPS" AS AN ENERGY TOOL

Most cars are designed to crumple on impact, front or back, because if they were rigid, the force of being hit would transfer into the passengers and cause damage. I think the Storymaker is designed to *give* that way too. When too many stories overwhelm us and build up pressure, we're designed to fall apart or fold. Falling apart (or folding in on ourselves) physically, emotionally, or mentally forces us to stop, pay attention, and make choices about how to proceed.

If you are one of those people who have chronic illness, frequent emotional collapse, ups and downs in your energies, or seem to catch every virus wafting by, you may want to play with how to relieve your Storymaker of pressure.

This silly little energy tool, given to me early on by my Councils, has probably saved my life multiple times. I call it the gas cap. It is like a pressure valve that I open to relieve excess stress, stories that don't serve me, or energies that are backing up and refusing to move.

Exercise: Adjusting Your Gas Caps

At your solar plexus, imagine there is a pressure valve, a round disk, with a handle you can grasp. In my mind's eye, it looks like an old-fashioned gas cap (see Figure 4.2)—nothing like the plug I use now on my electric car!

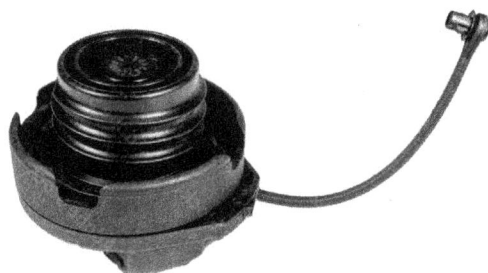

Figure 4.2. Gas Cap

Use your intuition to assess whether you need to relieve pressure by:

1. Loosening the cap (this will likely be the case most of the time),

2. Tightening the cap if you need to stop your fuel from leaking (this may happen on occasion), or

3. Reseating the cap for a better seal (this may occur, but only infrequently)

To relieve pressure: Grasp the handle, press in, and turn the cap *counterclockwise* (as if the clock is printed on your body). Like with a real gas cap, pressing in breaks the seal so you can unscrew it.

I don't generally unscrew it all the way, but I do turn it a bit, until I feel the pressure releasing from that area of my body. This usually stops my Storymaker from falling apart or galloping away with the narrative as well.

To stop energy leakage: Tighten the gas cap when you're leaking energy and can't seem to build up necessary pressure by pushing in and turning clockwise.

If it just feels wonky: Unscrew it all the way and reseat it to get a better seal.

Tip: The solar plexus area, or third chakra, is often a place where issues of identity in the world are stored. So it is a fruitful place to open your gas cap to relieve backed up energy in your Storymaker's creation of self. However, you can use this gas cap technique at any of your chakras and *anywhere else on your body* where you need to adjust pressure.

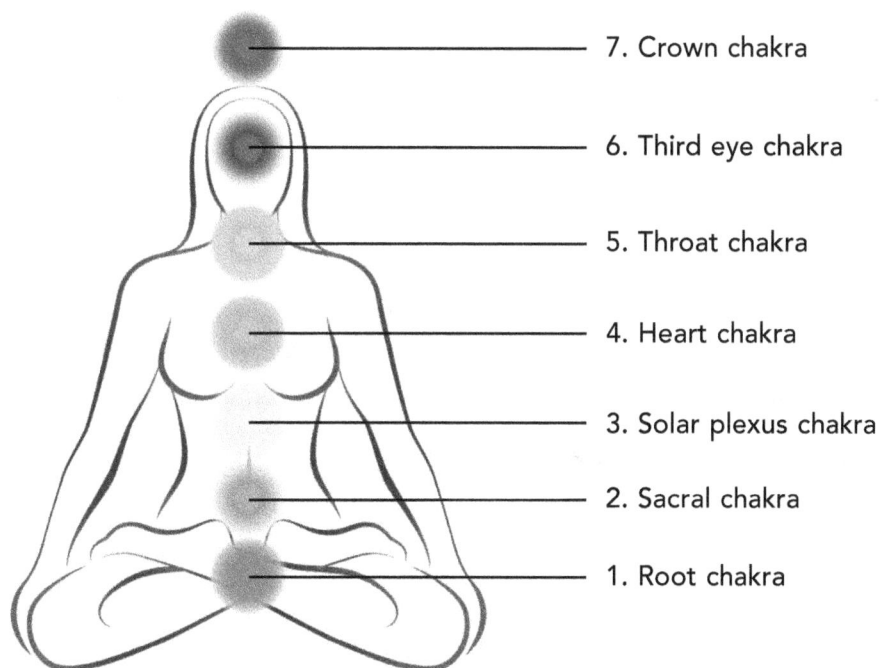

7. Crown chakra

6. Third eye chakra

5. Throat chakra

4. Heart chakra

3. Solar plexus chakra

2. Sacral chakra

1. Root chakra

Figure 4.3. Chakra Locations

Open a gas cap at your:

1. Root chakra for connecting with family, tribe, roots, the earth, and your creature nature. Loosen it if you feel disconnected from your roots. You can tighten it a bit if your sexuality is in overdrive, or if you feel too vulnerable to family—just remember to open it again as soon as possible, since this is where your "pilot light" sits that energizes all your chakras.

2. **Sacral chakra** for opening your access to your authentic self, your inner heart. I rarely tighten this one, but if you feel your essential self is under attack, you can batten down the hatches here.

3. **Solar plexus chakra** for identity, as I mentioned, and also for coping with the world. This area also influences how you process sound. You may need to experiment with how open or shut you want it, given what is happening around you. I sometimes close it down when someone is sliming me with toxic energy. But first I may have to loosen it to let my ire out!

4. **Heart chakra** for feeling shut down emotionally. Loosen it to release the bottleneck in your emotions. Similarly, you can tighten it a bit if you are flooded with too many feelings.

5. **Throat chakra** for communication challenges. If you are having trouble with speaking, loosen it. If the problem is compulsive speech, experiment with whether it helps to loosen or tighten it, or to pull it off and reseat the gas cap here.

6. **Third eye chakra** when you are either having trouble seeing or overwhelmed with vision. You can experiment with whether it helps to open or tighten the gas cap here when you can't sleep because your mind is racing.

7. **Crown chakra** to relieve spiritual stress or pressure built up in the brain. Experiment with whether you need to loosen or tighten it slightly if you feel you are being overwhelmed by cosmic forces, like sun flares.

ANCHORING FOR DIFFERENT PROCESSING TYPES

I mentioned in the introduction to this book that I suffer from sticky brain. This is an occupational hazard for people who tend to process information tonally—via sound, ears, or solar plexus. Information comes in and just gets stuck. *Tonal* is my main processor, and so my Storymaker is particularly vulnerable to incoming energies at my ears and solar plexus. I adjust gas caps at my ears and solar plexus frequently. It helps me release excess and modulate what comes in to me, cutting down on situations that used to flood me with too much information.

My Councils also taught me to use "touchstones" as first aid for my Storymaker. Touchstones are objects or words or thoughts that anchor us. In my case as a tonal, these are words or sounds that ground me. When I'm shopping, I often notice a song playing over and over in my head, and sometimes I'm even humming it. This helps me limit the information coming in by filling my tonal receptors with something I've chosen and find grounding.

There are four main processing types (tonal, visual, kinesthetic, and digital), and we all have all of them, though overwhelm often accrues via your primary or secondary one.

If you are primarily *visual*, you not only take in information mostly through your eyes, but also you steer according to vision, often inner vision. It can drive you crazy if others can't see what you *see*, perceive, or know in a higher way. So you will want to work with the gas caps at your third eye and root chakra. A touchstone for a visual is an image you can return back to again and again—often with symbolic significance, like a lotus. Or you can put your thumb out about eight inches in front of you (where you focus close), and alternate between looking at your thumb and looking at a distance. This helps your Storymaker regroup (and it relaxes your eyes).

If you are *kinesthetic*, meaning your information comes in through your feelings and whole body, you can adjust the gas caps at your heart and sacral chakras. When a kinesthetic gets overwhelmed, your Storymaker often just shuts down: You can't perceive any story. You go blank. Touchstones for kinesthetic processors include containers; swaddling yourself in a cloth or blanket or scarf is good. Also letting yourself feel, hold, or stroke something with texture or strong elements in it such as velvet, a stone with markings, or a carved figure can help.

If you are *digital*, meaning your trained brain is the main way that information enters your system and influences your Storymaker, then you can adjust gas caps on the bottoms of your feet or top of your head. Touchstone activities include doing math problems, puzzles, and calculations (e.g., figuring out a budget). When your brain shuts down or goes into over-thinky mode, you can bring your Storymaker back into balance by holding your feet or getting someone else to hold them for you.

CELTIC CLEARING

Unless you have been living on a desert island for the past many years, you have probably experienced that sense of being *slimed* by other people's energies, ideas, attitudes, politics, demands, entitlements, outrage, information, marketing, and bids for attention. Sometimes, it's more than a little sleep and avoidance can clear. One reason for this is that your Storymaker is designed to take in information from other people, from our shared culture, and integrate it into your creation of self. But we were not designed to process and slough off so much input. In short, most people's Storymakers are out of whack because of the acceleration of information coming at us from all sides.

The energy system your Storymaker uses to bring integration to your energies is what Donna Eden has called the "Celtic weave." If you see energies, it looks like a mass of interweaving, constantly moving figure eights and Celtic knots (interwoven figure eights with no beginning and no end), running through your entire energy field from the cellular level to the largest version of you. In her classic book, *Energy Medicine*, Donna describes the Celtic weave energy system as a:

> Living system, continually weaving new crossovers, ever expanding and contracting. . . . These crisscrossing energies permeating your body are the "connective tissue" of your energy systems. . . . The Celtic weave . . . laces through all your other energy systems and creates a resonance among them. It is a weaver of your force fields. It holds your entire energetic structure together. . . . *Like invisible threads* that keep all the energy systems functioning as a single unit, the Celtic weave networks throughout and around the body in spiraling figure-eight patterns.*

* Donna Eden with David Feinstein, *Energy Medicine: Balancing Your Body's Energies for Optimal Health, Joy, and Vitality* (Tarcher Penguin, 2008), 199–200.

This brilliant description of the Celtic weave energy system offers a potent visual for what my Councils define as the primary purpose of the Storymaker: to weave our energies into coherence to make meaning.

The Eden Method Celtic Weave exercise for reinstating your aura that I included as a final step in the Storymaker Reset protocol on page 91 is especially supportive of weaving us back together. But what happens if you need to first *clear* energies out that have infiltrated your field? The exercise, Celtic Clearing, offers first aid to deslime your field, to weed out other people's voices and perspectives and noise that have infiltrated your weaves. It also serves to retrain your Storymaker and Gatekeeper on what you do and don't want to include in the story.

Belinda, whose multiple breakups were followed by a diagnosis of auto-immune disease (lupus), found this exercise particularly helpful to clear out the rubble and strengthen her construction of self.

Exercise: Celtic Clearing

1. Start with the Celtic Weave exercise on page 93 to get your Storymaker's attention; the weaving energy will attune you to its nature.

2. Continue the Celtic weaving motion (see illustrations on page 94). You do not have to limit your weaves to the head, waist, knees, and ankles. Instead, you can make large and small weaves wherever they are needed around you or within you.

3. Focus on what you'd like to expel from your life, mind, or story (if you know it), and sharpen the outward motions of the weave so you are sweeping or pushing the unwanted energies out, out, out. If you have words, sounds, smells, colors, images that represent the "poisons" or toxins you wish to remove, you can say or invoke those as you do the clearing part of the figure eights.

4. As you inhale and bring your arms inward, soften your movements in toward the center, weaving integration in.

5. When you feel you have cleared out as much as you can for now, end

with the Eden Celtic Weave exercise, to reinforce the message to your Storymaker. You are giving it editorial instructions and supporting it overall.

* * *

Belinda used this exercise many times a day, whenever she was feeling her immune system flare and whenever she felt her sense of self-esteem cratering. She found it pulled her out of what she described as her Humpty Dumpty brokenness. She visualized replacing the broken eggshell from her "great fall" with a new, healthier egg, and doing Celtic Clearing was her way of caring for that egg—fighting off predators and bringing warmth to help it hatch.

HONEY

Around the time my Councils were preparing me to communicate with them by sending me metaphors, my dream life got considerably more interesting. This was true for daydreaming as well as for night dreaming. I spent a lot of time in bed that semester, just letting my mind wander. And, in retrospect, I think this was a crucial part of my awakening process, of opening to direct communication with my Councils. The realm of spirit is not linear, so learning to meander mentally is a valuable skill.

I had a dream at that time that was one of those aha dreams—recognition of a truth that changes everything eventually, even if at the time, it was just something I found amusing. I knew it was important without knowing why. In the dream, I saw that my body was not a solid self but was made up of nested selves. I saw those selves stream out of me at night, going all over the world, maybe all over the universe, to have different experiences. Then they came back every morning just before I was ready to wake up and nested within the form I was used to calling myself. And, in the dream, I realized I had access to all those selves, all those experiences, even if I hadn't been there as a whole self. I wrote a very bad poem about it called "My Body Is a Baklava."

The thing about baklava is that it requires honey to hold its layers together. And the thing about us is that we too require honey to hold our layers together. Those layers might be all the voices in you: your child self, inner critic, inner parent, best friend self, and the like. Those layers also include your past and counterpart selves, which I will talk about later in chapter 8. Those layers also include the selves you've dreamed and daydreamed and encountered in your imagination (and in the Country of the Mind). And they include the strata of your creation of self, roughly corresponding to levels in your chakras, which we'll explore later.

They all require honey to unify them into a single construction. In energetic terms, the Celtic weave system provides that honey. Whenever you trace figure eights and Celtic-weave patterns anywhere on your body or energy field, it activates the honey that holds you together. That is why people just starting to learn energy medicine techniques have found that they can help friends and family members tremendously just by figure-eighting their bodies and aura.

Sally, a beginning student of Eden Energy Medicine, reported on how she helped her father after his second knee-replacement surgery. His first had been a disaster. He had developed multiple infections and taken forever to heal. He was apprehensive about the second, but Sally, with all the confidence of one weekend class behind her, promised she'd help. So as soon as he came out of surgery, she figure-eighted all over his knee and his entire energy field, repeatedly. He recovered from this surgery with no infections and in record time.

This story is one of those anecdotal tales that don't prove anything scientifically, but Sally's father got what he needed, so he didn't need a scientific study to recognize that what she was doing felt good and seemed to help. Sally and her father both believed she had reduced his suffering: She brought some honey. As first aid, figure-eighting and Celtic weaving, done with love and in a spirit of trying to help, are a great go-to. Honey is generated whenever we bring to a situation love, kindness, energetic integration, our spiritual truth, or a story dynamic that allows energies to move in healthy ways. Science may not be able to isolate that in a lab, but in the lab of life, most of us can recognize how important this is when we or someone we encounter are short on honey.

There is a deeper aspect of this recognition that we need honey to hold us together. There is a tendency in our culture to want to describe energy in scientific terms, as moving molecules and atoms exchanging electrons and magnetic fields, and so forth. But the energies we are made of are more than the flattened, depersonalized nature science depicts. They are part of consciousness itself. And your body is not just a big energy machine; it is part of a big dance of consciousness communicating and creating meaning.

When we shift the paradigm this way, we can see how using figure eights, Celtic weaves, and bringing "honey" to communicate with your energies will directly influence how they move and form meaning. We can reclaim our power to heal ourselves and our loved ones using energy medicine, by recognizing that the energies we are made of communicate meaning and create a web of energy communication. This is true for the physical body, the mind, and the unity of mind-body-spirit.

Honey is what brings parts together into a unified whole; it brings energies together into a unified field. For you as an individual, it means that if you are falling apart, coming loose at the seams, or living stories that don't allow your spirit to learn and grow, you are probably short on honey.

Since we are collective beings, within our multiple dimensions of self and in our social connections, we need to learn good skills, in addition to figure-eighting and Celtic weaving, to increase the honey. Especially in this time when we are transitioning to a new level of consciousness, the stress of having so much Gatekeeper reactivity, so many power struggles, dries up the honey and makes it hard for anything to hold together in unified fields.

When Storymakers get overwhelmed, they stop producing the honey that holds us together. And that's one reason we become so vulnerable to other people's stories, to propaganda, and to conspiracy theories. We are not properly anchored and have lost our individual and social coherence.

Laughter brings honey. When you experience a moment of mirth, you increase the coherence within you. But that's not just any laughter—it is appreciative laughter. Making fun of someone else can dry out your honey. Similarly, when an audience laughs together at a comedian's jokes, when that comedian is bringing them to recognize their shared humanity, that is honey. When an audience bonds over nastiness, competition, high adrenaline, and power-over thinking, the honey dries out.

When a group hikes together harmoniously, honey is created, activating a unified field via feet and knee anchors. This usually does not happen on a forced march. Any shared work, shared endeavor, where individuals are contributing to a positive outcome, that increases the honey. A group of hooligans who bond over anger or destruction might feel solidarity, but their honey dries and their Storymakers falter.

The stories we choose as frames for our moment-by-moment existence can similarly bring the honey or destroy our coherence. In *Your Body Will Show You the Way*, I taught an exercise called Baklava Restoration. I'm bringing it back here to teach some variations you can use specifically to support your Storymaker to connect your layers of self. Try this when are not feeling coherent within yourself and need to glue yourself back together.

Exercise: Baklava Restoration with Variations

1. Stand about six to eight feet away from a wall, facing away, and invite all the layers of self to line up behind you.

2. Inhale, and as you exhale, very slowly back up, picturing each layer of self melding into you. When you run out of breath, stop, inhale, and on the next exhale, continue slowly backing up, gathering the layers into you.

3. When you reach the wall, use it as a bumper and put your hand back to cup your sacrum and tailbone (this is part of the steering mechanism of your Storymaker). Hold there for three to five seconds to seal the layers together.

4. When you feel them all glued together, trace a five-pointed star and circle on your sacrum to help the collation to hold. This star represents the balance

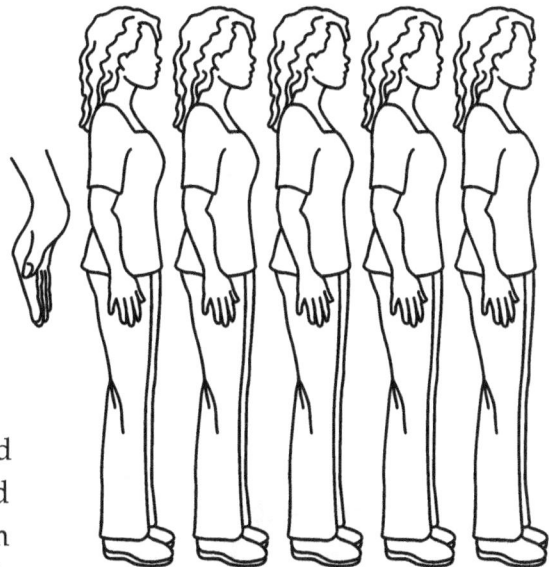

Figure 4.4. Baklava Restoration

of energies in many spiritual traditions and helps bring honey and balance everywhere within your construction of self. (See Figure 4.4B.)

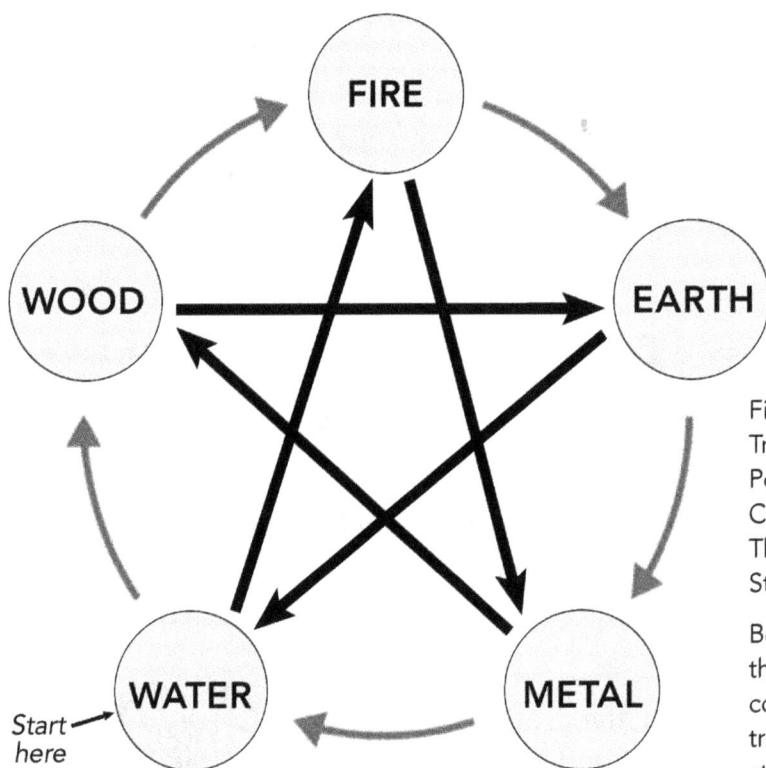

Figure 4.4B. Tracing the Five-Pointed Star and Circle (also called The Five-Element Star and Circle)

Begin with tracing the Water-Fire connection. After tracing the whole star, trace the circle.

Variation 1

As you back up and collect your layers, you can use a touchstone word that brings you honey such as "grace" or "acceptance"; you can sing a note that feels like *you*; or you can visualize a storyline that invites the layers in: maybe a welcome committee, pulling them home with a hug. These will help your Storymaker understand that you would like to bring more coherence to your energy dynamics. Even when you are not feeling like you have fallen apart, doing this exercise is a great way to communicate with your Storymaker about what kind of energy you want it to use to steer your ship. (We'll explore navigation more fully in chapter 7.)

The use of the movement and hold, together with bringing energetic honey, allows you to embody this intention and communication far more deeply and significantly than just visualizing or playing with touchstones on their own or just using a story that explains your connectedness. It ensures that your body gets the memo.

Once you have gathered the layers of self together and are holding your sacrum with one hand, you can use your other hand to anchor this communication into some of the Storymaker anchors: your knees, the arches of your feet, your Mingmen area, your heart, the sides of your face (hold one side at a time together with your sacrum), and your thinking cap (also, hold one side at a time together with your sacrum). This anchors the connection between selves into your Storymaker more firmly.

Variation 2

You can use this technique with other subsets of yourself to bring them onto the same page. For example, you can invite yourself at different ages to line up behind you and use the Baklava Restoration to bring more coherence between them and your present self: This helps heal your life story. Or you can call on your various subpersonalities to line up behind you—the serious you, the joker you, the needy you, the confident you, your inner critic, your inner cheerleader, and the like—and do the same action. This is a great way to heal your past selves by bringing the honey you've generated over the years to integrate them more positively into your construction of self.

Variation 3

Instead of lining up your multiple selves behind you, invite them to form a big figure eight around you, with your present, conscious self at the crossover point. This can include either your layers of self, your sub-selves, or even your past and future selves. If you are doing past and future selves, place the past selves on one side of the figure eight and future selves on the other.*

---

* Thanks to Paulette Taschereau and her Councils for this concept.

Then, send *honey*, like a wave, through the figure eight. You can get all these selves to figure-eight in unison, or hold hands and squeeze to pass the impulse around the figure eight, or sway with your bodies in a figure-eight motion (you are doing this while imagining the others joining in). You can also sing or dance to a song together, weave a web among you, or even sing up and down a scale together. You can laugh and send your mirth and joy circulating.

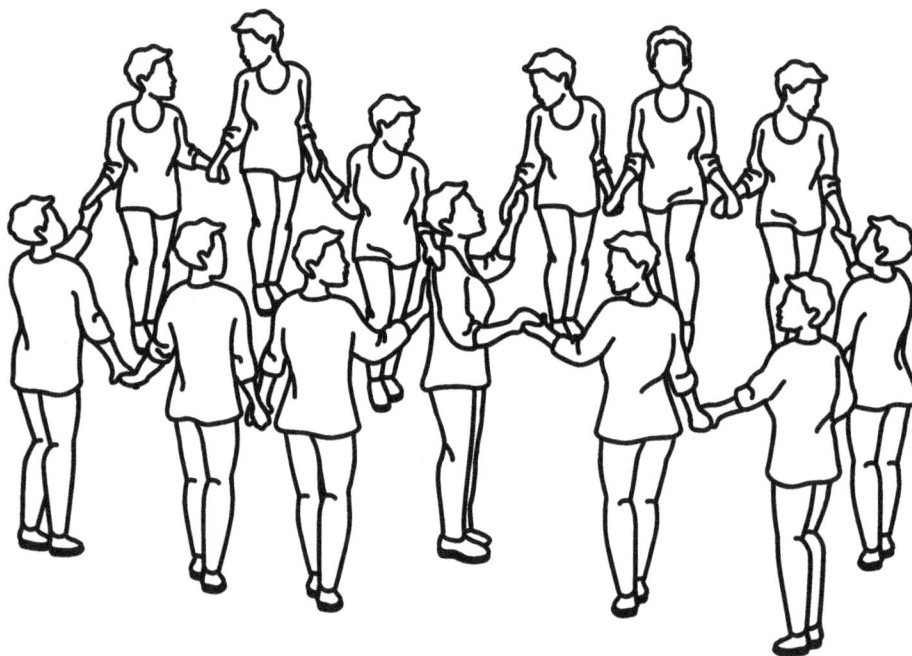

Figure 4.5. Diagram of Past and Future Selves in a Figure-Eight Formation

● ● ●

Honey, glue, communion, and presence bring coherence. They hold your dance of energies together. As you support your Storymaker by cultivating the honey, it will anchor you as an individual, deeply support your healing, and help heal our world.

ANTIDOTES

In witchy lore, wherever you find poison in nature, you find antidotes growing nearby. In this time when toxins are being spewed into our common discourse with fewer filters, it is useful to find and keep antidotes on hand.

First aid for a spider bite might include activated charcoal or antihistamines; for a snakebite, it is antivenom. First aid for your Storymaker involves anchoring and then seeking sanity. You can accomplish this by doing one or more of these strategies:

1. Focus on a "clean story" (one to replace the toxic narrative).

2. Reframe what is happening in ways that allow you agency.

3. Get yourself out of the situation and into a saner one.

4. Escape (for now) into a place in your mind or heart where the dynamics are wholesome for you.

An energy antidote is anything that counteracts the energy of the situation in a healthy way and gets your energies moving the way they are designed to move. If someone is being nasty, compassion is a great antidote. If they are being mean, kindness is a salve. If they are gaslighting you, affirming or celebrating some truth of your nature can help. If something is stuck, bringing gentle movement in can counteract the stuckness.

Herbalists often use essential oils or concoct salves or tinctures to preserve and "deliver" the antidotes. For energy work, simple energy medicine exercises, holds, and communications (like Reconciliation on page 8 or Consolation on page 71) can serve as antidotes. Touchstones, both physical and imaginary, can help you counteract toxins. Invoking a particular *flavor* of energy is helpful: Kindness has a certain vibration, so does peace, so does grace, and so does respect. You can say words that are kind, but without the energy of kindness, they mean nothing. On the other hand, meanness can be cloaked in a robe of logic or social expediency and still be toxic.

Anchoring involves using energy medicine to connect back into yourself. It also involves the skillful use of antidotes to counteract toxic effects when other people's influence overrides your ability to construct a life that has meaning and makes sense.

|||||||||||||||||| **Play with It!** ||||||||||||||||||

Visit each of your Storymaker anchors (or a subset of them) in any order you feel drawn to visit them: arches of your feet, knees, Mingmen area, heart chakra, sides of your face, and thinking cap.

Hold the anchor to establish contact, and then take a sounding (see page 32). You can ask, "Give me insight into [the influence of this person/this event/this story/this behavior] on my Storymaker."

Tune in to see what comes up for you. Remember, it might show up as words, images, direct knowing, a sound, sensation or feeling, a metaphor, a smell or taste, and so forth.

If you wish and have the time, you can enter that anchor as a doorway to explore where it leads you and what you find within it.

As you explore, ask yourself, "What is needed here? What antidote will detox what is distorting the healthiest truth here?"

- ◆ Sometimes the antidote is a symbolic action. For example, if you see cracks in the wall, you can call on the "Universal Support Team" to supply some energetic plaster to fill them in. (This is one way you can access energy resources—by asking a cosmic resource to bring what is needed and to help you with whatever is needed. I sometimes refer to them as the "Universal Supply Team" as well.)

- ◆ Sometimes the antidote is a literal action. For example, you see yourself hunched over and tight, and realize you need to gently stretch and unkink your muscles.

- ◆ Sometimes the antidote is a touchstone. For example, if you see yourself floating away, too light and blowing in the wind, you can hold a literal or imaginary stone while imagining the solidity of it filling you and helping you respond to gravity.

- ◆ Sometimes the antidote is honey—a need to bring kindness, laughter, and shared purpose to a situation.

- ◆ Sometimes the antidote is a reframe or shift in focus. You build a big box and put the troubling toxins into it and call the "Cosmic We-Haul" truck to remove it from your field. Or you recognize the purpose the troubling elements are serving and thank them for being teachers and awakeners. And you instruct your Storymaker to help your Gatekeeper recognize them as elements that need to be in the story for now.

Often you can bring an antidote by using an energy medicine exercise to rebalance the situation. You might hear a suggestion to do Expanding Hearts (see page 72). Keeping in mind the anchor where you took the sounding, do the suggested exercise—as a whole-body exercise or in miniature right there on the anchor place.

Here's an example:

> I want to find out how following the news about war in the Middle East is affecting my Storymaker. I hold both sides of my face and ask, "How is my following news about the Middle East affecting my health and well-being?" I see a long line of my Jewish ancestors and feel the pain of the various pogroms and diasporas they've lived. I feel them pulling at me, making their stories my story.
>
> I put them into a big figure eight, with all of them on one side, me in the middle, and on the other side, I put my future selves and a bunch of people from our extended family who have thrived after being transplanted to new soil. We do Variation 3 of the Baklava Restoration together. I invite the future selves to each contribute some honey to send through the figure eight back to our ancestors.
>
> Each of them in turn says something like "I learned resilience. I am whole, and I give you my hand." They then send a squeeze around the circle,

gifting resilience around the eight. As it passes through me, I fill my body with that gift, that quality. Resilience, forgiveness, self-sufficiency, humor, each in turn circulate and strengthen both me, and the collective of souls gathered in the eight.

At the end, we each thank one another for our contributions to the world. And I take a few minutes to hold each of the other Storymaker anchors to bring the qualities shared to all parts of my Storymaker.

● ● ●

Whenever I feel myself going out of balance, emotionally, energetically, and/or physically, I turn first these days to holding my Storymaker anchors. I hold my knees while watching the news, I cradle my face when I'm reading an email from a friend that strikes me wrong, or I hold my thinking cap to reclaim my mind when my brain is galloping away with it! It is amazingly effective in restoring me to myself.

If we are not anchored into our Storymaker, then we are at the mercy of other people's Storymakers. And, in this day and age, when our inboxes and feeds and ears are full of the noise of other people's agendas, anchoring is a crucial first step in healing any ailment of body or mind.

It is important to remember in this very complicated time that simple solutions—antidotes, a little honey, a touchstone, releasing pressure by unscrewing a gas cap, and the like—can keep us sane. Coming home to ourselves is powerful medicine.

CHAPTER FIVE

Terms of Engagement

My friend has a very quiet head. We'll be driving somewhere, and I'll ask, "What are you thinking?" She'll reflect for a moment and say, "Nothing." And she means it. She's quiet in there. She doesn't usually remember her dreams and when she does, she never knows anyone in them. She's someone whose Storymaker is firmly anchored and seated in her body. It makes her calm and present, unflappable. She doesn't speak unless she has something she needs to say. Fascinating concept.

I, on the other hand, make up for it with lots of speech and too many stories. When we are out and about, each person I see comes with a story. My mind automatically tries to explain who they are and why they're there doing what they're doing. It is endlessly entertaining—and often exhausting.

My Councils have frequently had to help me declutter my mind and body when the stories, news, and what-ifs tie my energies in knots. They tell me, "Take a deep breath. There is no past. There is no future. There is only this moment." They repeat it over and over, as I breathe deeply, in through my nose and out through my mouth. It calms me to drop the stories from the past and the ones about the future and just be here in the empty present.

Try it and see what it feels like. I find it both consoling and somewhat disconcerting. "What?" my Storymaker asks. "Abandon all the glorious, interesting stories, all my fantasies about the future and revisiting of the past? All the knowledge filling my brain?" Then, it calms. I imagine that's what my quiet friend feels much of the time.

At the retreat center I used to visit twice a year, the outhouse had a sign at eye level, presumably designed to help us overcome the stink. It said, "No self, No problem." It was another mantra that basically says, "Drop it." Like getting a dog to let go of the ball and calm down so you can re-engage: Drop it.

But, alas, I rarely stay here in the quiet, in the here and now. My Wiser Self is a member of several Councils that practically guarantee my talking self will be on the move. And by nature, by the terms of engagement I chose as a soul, I am a messenger, a storyline tracker, traveling between worlds.

FRAMING

Each of us is a unique instrument; it is useful to know who you are. Setting the terms of engagement and cultivating a Storymaker that truly serves you is not about following some rules *out there* on how to become a certain kind of person. It is about understanding how you are, recognizing how you frame your reality at all levels of your being, and learning to support your nature with appropriate nurture.

When my Councils say, "There is no past, there is no future, there is only this moment," they are helping me come home and reset my Storymaker by radically shifting the instructions I am giving to my body. They are setting the terms of engagement back to ground zero.

Your body lives in the now. Your mind doesn't. And that creates a basic problem: Your stories and *talking self* are taking you into all kinds of territory beyond your physical reality, and since your body lives your stories, how does it know which stories to embody? How does it remember where you are, how to navigate, and what is required for safety? How does your mind discern reality and truth that is grounded in your own lived experience that is relevant to the instrument *you* are?

The equipment for discerning truth and grounding in lived experience is built into your body, into your Storymaker and Gatekeeper. That's why your consciousness needs these mechanisms. They create and run the auto-pilot that operates most of your body and mind functions. They allow your consciousness and mind to travel but also secure the sanctity of your earth elemental self.

Because we have this equipment, healing and being well means learning to work with it in support of the kind of being you are.

Remember when I asked you in chapter 1 what your soul feeds are? Your soul feeds reflect your deeper purpose. A bridge builder needs very different equipment than a stargazer. A trickster trains their Storymaker and Gatekeeper to function differently than a peacemaker would. But at least one thing is true for most of us: When the mind is off adventuring in fantasies, in thinking, or in other people's stories and beliefs, we are denatured, decontextualized, and our earth elemental selves can't navigate and function for long.

Periodically throughout the day, it is helpful to come home and reset your Storymaker and calm your Gatekeeper. Drop the ball and commit once again to your home base. Much of the energy medicine in this book will serve to reset your Storymaker and calm your Gatekeeper, including the exercise Coming Home on page 46, the variations of the exercise Consolation on page 71, and particularly holding any or all of the Storymaker anchors introduced on page 91. In addition, here are some simple energy medicine tools that help reset you to ground zero when your stories pull you off-center.

Protocol: Acrobat's Pole, Torus Pole, Yin-Yang Pole

Just as the earth revolves around an axis, your body has an axis of "now," "here," and inner/outer balance. Each of these can be worked with individually, but it is useful to adjust all three axis poles to help bring you into presence.

Acrobat's Pole

Acrobat's Pole gets its name from the balancing pole used to balance an acrobat on the high wire. However, in this case, the pole runs horizontally front to back through your solar plexus. It represents your experience of the timeline. In front of you is future; behind you is past. When you are trapped in anticipation or reliving memories (and resentments) or just feeling out of sync, this is an important tool for adjusting back to *now*.

1. Imagine the pole extending in front of you and behind you, through your solar plexus. Grasp it with one hand behind and one hand ahead of you.

2. Like an acrobat, intuitively using the pole for balance, gently pull the pole forward and back until you find the *now* position.

3. Hold the pole there for the count of three deep breaths, and then trace a five-pointed star and circle (see page 110) on your solar plexus to help your Storymaker remember this balance point.

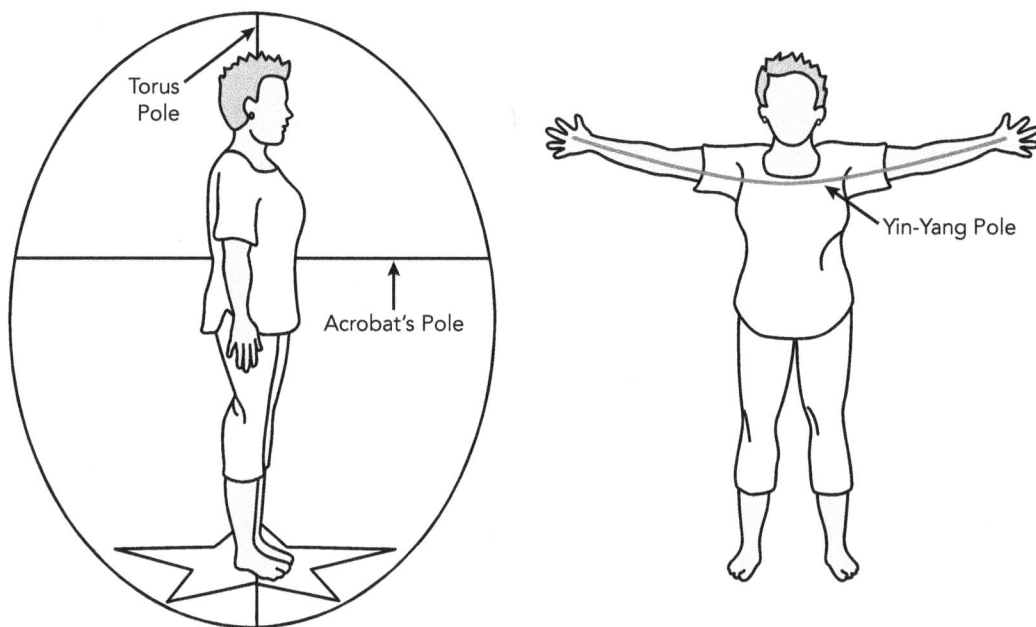

Figure 5.1. Acrobat's Pole, Torus Pole, Yin-Yang Pole

Torus Pole

The Torus Pole runs vertically, extending above you through the crown of your head and below you down through your root and into the ground. It is your axis of place, of *here*. If you are feeling disoriented, displaced, or not present in some way, this is a tool to bring you back.

1. Grasp the pole above your head a few inches above your crown. If you wish, you can also grasp it below at your root. But since it is uncomfortable for many people to reach both positions, it is sufficient to adjust

this pole one-handed from above. This is the portion of your pole that represents the heavens, aspirational energy. The portion of the pole extending down from your roots represents grounding, earth-based energy.

2. Gently move the pole upward and downward until you intuitively feel it settle into your *here* point.

3. Hold the pole there for the count of three deep breaths, and then trace the five-pointed star and circle (see page 110) on your crown to help hold the pole in this new position.

Yin-Yang Pole

Your Yin-Yang Pole runs through the center of your chest and out each arm. It helps you balance your receptive realms (yin) with your active realms (yang). This pole is extremely flexible.

1. Extend your arms fully with your palms facing forward. Feel the pole extending left (yin) and right (yang).

2. Grasp the pole with your hands and pull it left and right to get it centered.

3. When you feel a balance point, open your palms, and Celtic-weave the area at least three times (see page 93).

4. End with both hands on your heart chakra. This anchors integrated yin and yang, inner and outer focus, into your Storymaker.

End this protocol with a full-body Celtic Weave to reinforce the messaging to your Storymaker, your entire mind, about where presence, ground zero, lives in your body.

• • •

Mindy sought energy medicine help after her seventh car accident, when she slammed into a car in front of her, not noticing it had stopped, and ended up with her fourth concussion. Her friends told her that she was such a space cadet and shouldn't continue to drive if she couldn't do something about her spaciness.

She didn't remember a time when her mind was clear. And now, after seven crashes, Mindy lived with widespread chronic physical pain as well.

She grew up in a house with two alcoholic parents. While her father tended to just withdraw from the world when he was drinking, her mother would fall into shame and blame behaviors. She would blame Mindy's father for her drinking and for everything she forgot to do, and she would shame the kids when they complained or needed something from her.

Mindy's response to the chaotic ups and downs was to disappear into a fog state, similar to her father. Throughout her childhood, she frequently sprained her ankles, banged her knees, and bumped her head because she just wasn't there, in her body, paying attention. Likewise, she was neither reliving her past nor looking toward a better future. She was emotionally blank much of the time and most comfortable when people were not focused on her. Despite this, her friends cared about her and often mothered her, reminding her to eat and to take care of herself.

As Mindy grew up, her Storymaker basically resisted making stories and setting terms of engagement. She saw life as just too unpredictable to allow her to have dreams or hopes. Her friends had encouraged her to get into therapy to clear out the damage from her childhood. But despite years of therapy, which gave her insights into why she was spacey and helped her get in touch with some of the emotional trauma, she couldn't seem to get the clouds to lift. She felt like the spaciness was just programmed into her body.

And she was right. The Storymaker and the Gatekeeper are both programmable, designed to learn and codify our learning. Mindy had learned to space out as a part of forming a self. She needed to create a new self that could handle presence. And she needed to teach her Storymaker and Gatekeeper to embody the new truth. It reminded me of the phenomenon some alcoholics experience. It's not enough to stop drinking and understand why you were drinking. You sometimes have to go back and learn the life skills you didn't learn when you were drunk.

Since Mindy was not really in her body, when we tried having her hold her Storymaker anchors nothing happened. There was no sensation in her at all. She could barely feel her hands on her knees, back, feet, and so forth. This was an indication that she needed to adjust her poles first, to come into the here and now on the same page with her body. But when she tried to grasp her Acrobat's Pole, it came apart in her hands, like one of those collapsing canes with elastic holding the parts together.

We both found this telling: After so many collisions, her Storymaker had come up with a creative solution. It just let go on impact, even when the touch was friendly and well-meaning.

Mindy had to actually start by reassembling her Acrobat's Pole and Torus Pole. She worked from the center, aligning the pieces and fusing them with Radiance, using the Divine Hook-Up: She plugged her left finger into the heart of the Divine and used her other hand to bring Radiance to supply the glue. Then she was able to get her poles adjusted. And once this happened, the lights turned on in her eyes. She could hold her Storymaker anchors and feel them grounding her into her body, use the exercise Coming Home on page 46 to bring her out of the fog repeatedly during the day, and then turn her attention to clearing the clouds out of her body's memory banks and creating a new story.

As a first step, Mindy used her Acrobat's Pole to help her show up for herself and cultivate presence at different ages.

Your axis poles can be used for balance and also to help you travel within the dimensions of yourself. You can travel backward in consciousness along the back portion of your Acrobat's Pole, for example, to visit parts of your past. Or you can travel forward along the front portion of the pole to gain insights into your future.

Try this: Travel back along the pole until you find a place where you intuitively want to pause. If you can reach it physically, grasp the pole there. Otherwise, just tune in with your consciousness to that portion of the pole. Take a sounding there (see page 32). Open to getting images, sensing presence, hearing something, feeling, smelling, tasting, and knowing directly.

You can ask in that place, "What age are you?" You may see a version of yourself, a vague figure, or something symbolic. You may just hear a voice telling you an age. Even if you hear or sense nothing, just continue conversing.

Ask, "What can you tell me about your story?" You may hear a response, see an image, have a thought pop into your head, feel a sensation or emotion, or again draw a blank. Lovingly trace with your hands the outline of the self you find there or what you imagine to be its outline.

Adjust the Acrobat's Pole for that version of yourself. Celtic-weave the figure to help it find integration, and then continue back along the pole to find other places where you intuitively feel called to stop and interact. Then, when you feel done, return back to the "now point" within your solar plexus, check to make sure your Acrobat's Pole is still adjusted, then Celtic-weave your body in small and large weaving motions. End with both hands on your heart.

This is a wonderful way to visit parts of yourself along the timeline and bring healing and support to your Storymaker.

Note: In case you were wondering, yes, you can also travel along the Torus Pole to explore your orientation to the heavens and earth, and along the Yin-Yang Pole to work with habits relating to where your focus gets stuck or blocked. All three of these support dimensional travel and conversations with dimensions of yourself.

DISCERNMENT

Mindy had sleepwalked much of her life and didn't trust her judgment. Given how skewed her parents' perceptions had been when she was growing up, it was reasonable for her to doubt her own thoughts and understanding of things. She often relied on friends to guide her and keep her on track. And she often ended up recognizing truth only when she bumped into it somehow, like walking into walls to determine where the room ends.

Discernment is a big issue for lots of us these days. Not only has black-and-white, polarized thinking and tribalism been on the rise, making it hard to parse the truth of passionately held but conflicting perspectives, but also the overwhelming volume of information has caused many of us to experience dysfunction in our Storymakers—in our perceptions of truth, our handle on reality and fact, and our ability to anchor our thinking in common sense and experience.

Mindy realized she needed to develop better judgment and more clarity. She wanted to know if energy medicine could help her with that. It definitely could. Her most important step, as she discovered, was to come home to her instrument of perception: her body. In her vague state, she couldn't use her Storymaker to make coherent meaning.

After that, it was something of a circular process, not a sequence:

She learned to tune her instrument for greater receptivity. That's partly achieved through getting the instrument working properly and partly achieved by learning to communicate with her own being over and over again, using the language of energy. She needed to form a bonded relationship with her instrument.

She worked to evolve her Storymaker and Gatekeeper to address where they had been damaged growing up and as a result of her car accidents. Without reworking them, she'd always be living inadequate storylines *and* reacting to them—in her case, with fog.

She was also able to use techniques I'm teaching in this book to clear the habits that came from having to live stories that did not allow her to be safe and thrive. This went beyond clearing trauma. She needed to address the ways she'd learned to disconnect in the face of other people's energies. She needed to get to know what her own beautiful mind-body-spirit instrument was capable of.

Throughout the process, she kept discovering her agency: the creative self who could choose and write the stories she was living.

Although this was a long process, which included healing her body's damaged musculoskeletal system, it was a process that didn't require her to wait until the end to feel good. It was more a journey of discovery than one of recovery. The Storymaker, even a broken one, is often quite responsive to small efforts. Mindy discovered her body and mind supported her efforts to speak energy and showed her what they needed moment by moment.

Discernment combines the ability to sort through information and to choose what is relevant and nourishing.

Wisdom involves being able to frame the situation and make choices that allow you, and hopefully others, to thrive.

Mindy was so spacey much of the time that she was not great at perceiving, at bringing information in. She was so programmed to avoid judgment that she had trouble sorting her experience and recognizing what was relevant for her. And although she showed a capacity for wisdom in choosing a few reliable friends and allowing them to help her, she was easily swayed by unreliable people when her friends weren't around to help.

One friend taught her to use a pendulum when she had to make a choice and no one was around to help her decide what to do. She was quite dependent on it, frequently pulling it out to ask for guidance, rather than trying to gather information another way. The problem with a pendulum, which can be helpful in amplifying body knowing, is that it is not wise. It uses a simplistic vocabulary of yes-no that wipes out nuance and rarely gets us to our truth.

Using her Yin-Yang Pole offered Mindy a new "amplifier"—a new way to activate discernment and get more dimensional insight. The axis runs through the heart chakra, a Storymaker anchor and home of energies related to connection: how we relate to others and the world around us. And it runs along the bottoms of each arm, encompassing two energy flows (heart meridian and small intestine meridian in traditional Chinese medicine). My Councils call them the "heart/connection" and "choice/discernment" streams.

This simple Rabbit Ears technique gave Mindy a more robust tool for bringing in insight and sorting truth. It is named after the old-fashioned antenna people used to use to adjust reception on their TV sets.

Exercise: Rabbit Ears

1. To activate your antennae, balance your Yin-Yang Pole by extending your arms and grasping the ends of the pole with your hands, pulling gently left and right until you find a balance point in the center. Celtic-weave this pole three times (weaving across your chest), ending with both hands on your heart.

2. Now, trace along the inner edge of your arm (in line with your little finger), starting at each armpit and stroking along the bottom, inner edge of your arm out to your little finger. Repeat this on the other side. This activates your heart/connection stream.

3. Next, trace back up along your arm on the outer edge, from little finger up onto your shoulder. Dip back a few inches toward your shoulder blades, then continue tracing up the side of your neck to your cheekbone, and over to end at the opening of your ear. Repeat on the other side. This activates your choice/discernment stream. By tracing these energy streams, you are activating energies that support connection and wisdom (heart/ connection stream) and discernment (choice/discernment stream).

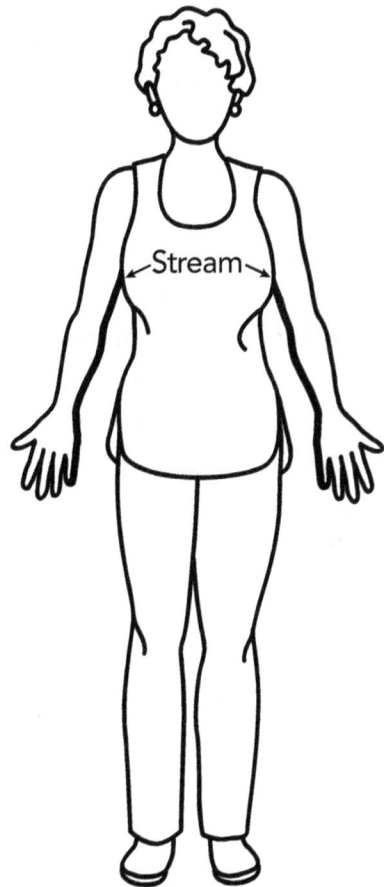

Figure 5.2.
Heart/Connection Stream

4. Now, put your arms up in a V position, like a rabbit ear antenna. Ask for insight or information about something, as you do when taking soundings. And then twist and turn your rabbit ear antenna every which way until you feel like you are getting the clearest reception. (Note, these antennas are bendy, not rigid.)

Jot down whatever comes to you in response to your questions. Remember, open-ended questions yield better, more nuanced insight. And, for the next few days, test that information to see how it matches other data, evidence, and the perspectives of friends you trust.

Note: The Yin-Yang Pole isn't a right-answer machine. It helps amplify your perceptions so you can develop wisdom. It is meant to provide more robust insight and information, not tell you what to think!

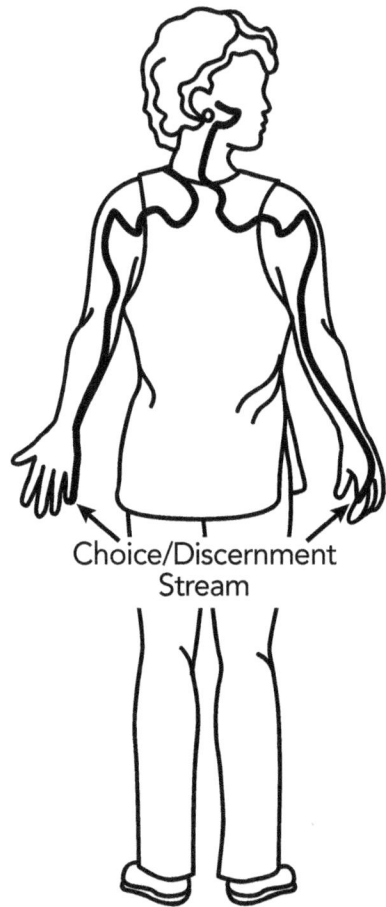

Choice/Discernment Stream

Figure 5.3.
Choice/Discernment Stream

• • •

As Mindy had to learn, discernment isn't a yes-no proposition. Because being present was a pleasant change from switching off (mostly), she enjoyed exploring all kinds of ways she could switch on again. She had a strong spiritual belief system, so it felt natural to her, as she learned new habits, to use these strategies:

1. Seek inner guidance.

2. Frame a situation appropriately.

3. Build on her spiritual beliefs as she learned to gather information.

4. Test it against inner knowing, outer validation, or evidence.

5. Recognize what was happening, what was still needed, and what the implications were for all people involved.

And, as she pursued this process, which she called her spiritual curriculum, she was amazed to see her bones and muscles heal unbelievably quickly. She recovered her structural integrity along with the repair of her Storymaker, and it freed her from the chronic pain.

DIMENSIONS OF STORY

At any given moment, most of us are living multiple stories. We have the "official story" in our mind of what is happening right now. We have the backstory of what it means in the larger scheme of things. We have the future and past stories that impinge on our now. We have the larger contexts that impact our ability to set terms of engagement. And that doesn't begin to capture the myriad ways stories from other people and media contribute moment by moment to creating our reality, perceptions, and experience.

For example, I am outside in my yard planting a vegetable garden. We have *character* (me), *plot* (I'm planting a vegetable garden), and *setting* (my yard). We have the *meaning* of it: I want to feel more self-sustaining. I want to be able to make a salad from what I grow. We have the factors that influence the plot, character, and setting: I need more exercise (*motive*), I want to be closer to nature (another *motive*), I have never succeeded with plants in the past because I hate getting my hands dirty (*backstory*), most of my friends have gardens and I'm experiencing FOMO—fear of missing out (*plot thickener*). In my head, a *voice* is narrating the experience, telling me I'm out of shape (*internalized storyline* from past), and another voice is wondering how long I have to do this before I can go read my book (*sub-character* in head). In between these moments, a story from the newspaper is impinging on my energies. I'm worrying about climate change and whether we have a will in our country to do something about it.

Overall, my body is living considerably more story than just the simple acts of digging holes and planting seeds!

Before falling into an overly complex analysis of story, I would just say: Your body lives your stories, plural—past, present, future, and imaginary—and the stories of the people who influence you, the stories of your world and times, and the stories of your own unique soul. And although you can fight story with story (like fighting fire with fire), by analyzing and reworking the narratives that guide your life, it is useful to be able to drop beneath the storylines and work with the Storymaker directly.

For example, yesterday I read an article about becoming more conscious of self-talk and learning to turn negative self-talk into something more positive. My Councils used to do something similar in my training. I came from a family that was very critical, always pointing out where someone or something (including me) was falling short of perfection. That was a terrible habit my Storymaker and Gatekeeper had to unlearn. I would see someone and what would pop into my mind was some kind of critique or judgmental observation. My Councils said, "Whenever you notice this, stop and choose to identify one good thing you notice about them."

I really enjoyed the One Good Thing game. They were basically inviting me to apply an antidote to the situation. And it helped. At some point, I noticed when I'd meet someone new, I'd automatically fall into One Good Thing (and its sequel: One More Good Thing). This would often drown out the negativity. Until I forgot about it. And slowly I found myself falling back into Several Critical Things.

Despite months of vigilance, the habits seemed to be too deeply ingrained, programmed somewhere that wasn't touched by the antidotes. I noticed this was true of any habit I tried to change. I could change the behavior for a while, sometimes for months or a year, but then once I stopped being vigilant, the old habits would re-emerge.

I realized that although it can help to talk story to story, it helps more to work on the energetic level to rewrite the story. To clear the negativity at its source, I had to travel within to locate the *templates of experience,* programmed into my Storymaker and Gatekeeper, that basically had me propping myself up by putting others down. I had to clear those templates and implant new ones; I had to reprogram my Storymaker.

I call this process Storyline Track and Balance because it involves chasing down where the story lives in your energy anatomy and balancing it energetically. It also involves traveling within the dimensions of self to work with your energies where they live. We are multi-dimensional beings, and when you can access those places within yourself, you can participate in writing (and healing) the stories you live where they are stored, in the dimension of self they emanate from, in consultation with your deepest truth.

What Is Your Storyline?

- ◆ Your storyline is made up of the conscious and deeper narratives that guide how the energies of your body, mind, and spirit behave.

- ◆ The storyline is coded into templates: energy maps or blueprints that direct your multiple energies in what to do and when and how to do it.

- ◆ Your Storymaker forms the templates and storyline, often in collaboration with your conscious mind. And your Gatekeeper is charged with keeping those templates and allocating energies based on the instructions coded into them.

- ◆ The storyline and templates can also be influenced by how you think, live, experience things, and interpret your experiences, as well as by input from others and from your environment.

This process of experiencing—learning from experience and codifying that learning to guide future experience—is woven into us at all levels of our being.

We are not a new person every moment. We build up a composite energy map over time of templates and instructions that guide our autopilot. And, sometimes, those maps are so strong, they can be hard to override when we want to steer the ship in another direction. Sometimes they conflict with one another and steer the ship in circles or break the equipment.

You might be wondering, *Isn't this just a fancy way of saying the brain stores experience in memory and guides the functions of the body?* That is the belief in our culture. But I don't subscribe to the brain-on-a-stick view of our amazing being. If we are indeed a swirl of energies, energies with consciousness, then the mechanism of learning has to be built into our whole mind, our whole self, in all the places it lives. And what can be learned can be unlearned, augmented, reshaped, and revised to support our individual and collective evolution.

While reprogramming the brain can help shift a storyline, it does not always reach the other parts of us where the storyline lives and where it influences our feelings, choices, body functions, and energy allocation.

If you are familiar with energy psychology tapping (aka EFT), in which the person calls to mind an emotional issue, fear, or habit, and taps on various acupuncture points to quickly clear the habits, you can understand that memory, habits, and beliefs reside in your energy systems, not just in the brain.

Storyline is more than just the narrative of events in your head. It is the pattern that guides your choices and actions and your very functioning. And it is a pattern that is written in the language of energy and stored in various places within your multi-dimensional self.

We all form these patterns, which may include multiple templates of encoded experience and learning. And they will, for the most part, keep the ship on course.

For example, you may have, over time, developed a storyline about yourself as a peacekeeping, mediator type of person. This could arise from experience or from recognition of your soul feeds and individual nature. When conflict arises, you instinctively or consciously see it as your job to step in and try to keep the peace. You behave in line with that narrative much of the time, and when you can't, you probably feel guilty or disturbed that you were not able to mediate and make a difference. Your Gatekeeper enforces the storyline and fuels it, unless there are individual templates that say it is not safe to live it.

If you are another kind of a person who has created a storyline to "live and let live," you might see the same conflict and instinctively move away. In your programming, it is not your job to intervene with the conflict, and when you don't intervene, you feel aligned with your truth and probably feel positive that you avoided getting caught up in the conflict. In this case, your Gatekeeper is enforcing and fueling a different storyline.

Your storyline lives and expresses itself on many levels. Consider it from the everyday dimension down into your deepest identity:

- On the surface level, you have the life circumstances that appear to define you: You live in a cultural context, have taken on certain roles, have stated and unstated goals or aspirations, and have affiliations dictated by your birth and family and by your own actions over the years. You have a physical body that expresses itself with physical symptoms and sensations.

- On a deeper level, you have a self-image and carry beliefs about who you are and aren't. This self-image can be seen as a kind of composite map of "you" that represents your experiences in this life—both within yourself and in response to interactions with others.

- Beneath that, you have your own nature dictating your interpretations. Many cultures have ways to understand our natural elements: your astrological profile, your balance of elements such as water-wood-fire-earth-metal in traditional Chinese medicine, your processing type (tonal, visual, digital, or kinesthetic), your Enneagram number, and so forth—all reflect your deeper nature, who you know yourself to be. These aspects of your being are coded into your body and nervous system, and shape how you encounter experience right from the beginning.

- Beneath that, you have a composite self made up of all your multiple lifetimes and counterpart selves. Some of those agendas and experiences can bleed through and color your experiences and understandings of this lifetime, particularly in the early years, when you are laying down templates to guide your reality of this lifetime. (If multiple lifetimes is a bridge too far for you, think of your many life phases as lifetimes, and the many aspects of your personality as your counterpart selves.) The truth of this dimension is the need to form a composite that allows you to function as your circumstances change!

◆ Beneath that is your larger nature—what I refer to as your Wiser Self— the part of you that has created the body-mind-spirit matrix of *you* in this life as an instrument on which to play the music of your being. At this level, what I think of as the Council level because it's where I meet up with my Councils, you have a deeper nature and truths that fuel certain types of efforts and aspirations and don't particularly support others.

At the Wiser Self level of your narrative, your individual truth is interrelated with collective narratives. Therefore, you may know yourself to be part of larger movements and larger purposes. These may or may not be apparent to others viewing your life, but they do provide inner guidance about your deeper truth.

◆ Beyond all of this is a kind of cosmic narrative, of which we sometimes can get indications via the behaviors of the cosmos and our own intuitive imaginative receptors.

What Is Your Storyline from Your Spirit's Perspective?

It is sometimes helpful to turn that whole understanding upside down and ask, "From the perspective of my spirit, what is my storyline?" Different aspects of this multi-level self can be found stored at various levels of the chakras. These spinning whirling energies both store energy templates and carry energies from level to level within us, and from source to world and back.

◆ On the largest level, your storyline is your karmic truth and path. It is the *kind* of being or instrument you are. It is the inner intention, guiding myth, and deeper purpose. (Levels 6 and 7 of the chakras.) Things that align with your larger purpose get energized, and things that conflict with that purpose are usually blocked or resisted.

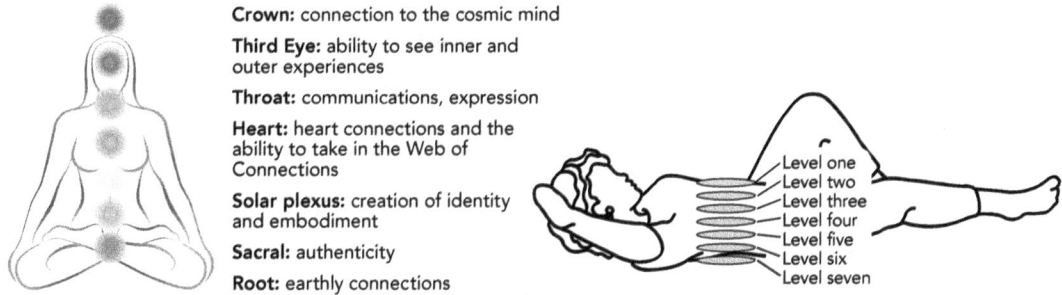

Crown: connection to the cosmic mind

Third Eye: ability to see inner and outer experiences

Throat: communications, expression

Heart: heart connections and the ability to take in the Web of Connections

Solar plexus: creation of identity and embodiment

Sacral: authenticity

Root: earthly connections

Level one
Level two
Level three
Level four
Level five
Level six
Level seven

Figure 5.4. Energetic Priorities of the Seven Chakras and Levels of Self

- We have a storyline that gets set up as contracts before we are born—agreements or intentions to enact certain dramas or explore certain themes. (Level 5 of the chakras.)

- We have a storyline that gets set up as our childhood unfolds—family patterns, learned habits, beliefs, and expectations we set up to encode our reality. And there's also the plot and identity of our life. What we believe happened to us, what we believe about what we've done, and what we tell ourselves and others about who we are and how we are. (Level 4 of the chakras.)

- And at another level, there is the ongoing drama—who we live with, who we believe ourselves to be right now, and what we are striving to be. (Levels 2 and 3 of the chakras.)

- And on the surface, influencing the ongoing drama, there is the body's chemistry and symptoms of ease and dis-ease, comfort and discomfort—which is where Western medicine usually tries to track the storyline and sometimes comes up short! (Level 1 of the chakras.)

Since your storyline guides the operations of your body and frequently of your mind as well, it is useful to know how to track it *where it lives*. We'll explore many ways to do this in coming chapters. But, for an initial dip, try this guided visit down into a single chakra: your solar plexus chakra. This chakra often stores energy dynamics related to your creation of identity, embodiment of your identity, and ways of coping with the world around you.

Mindy used this process repeatedly in her quest to learn what she felt and perceived. By going inward and taking soundings, she found it took the pressure off her to *know* and gave her space to just let the parts of herself show up and reveal themselves to her.

In this visit, we're not necessarily focusing on clearing templates (that comes in chapter 8) but on experiencing what it is like to take soundings in various dimensions of our being. However, since energy medicine is always about communication and dialogue, feel free to bring in antidotes, energy medicine tools, exercises, and gifts, or ask for help from guides at each location.

Guided Visit: Taking Soundings in Your Dimensions of Self

To get the most out of the guided visits in this book, you can either record the text for yourself, leaving silent spaces to allow yourself to explore as guided, or you can download an MP3 recording I've provided and use that. See page 13 for instructions on how to access the MP3s.

In this visit, we're going to explore the levels of one single chakra, your third, or solar plexus chakra, to take soundings with a particular storyline or issue in mind. Place one hand on your solar plexus chakra and your other hand on your heart chakra. Breathe in through your nose and out through your mouth for at least three slow, deep breaths.

Now, keeping your hand on your solar plexus, move your other hand down to your second, or sacral chakra, between your pubic bone and your belly button. Again, breathe in through your nose and out through your mouth for at least three slow, deep breaths. Bringing in the chakras on either side is like shoring up a hole you are digging so it doesn't collapse.

Now continue to hold your solar plexus with one hand, but remove your other hand from your sacral chakra. In general, you will keep one hand on the solar plexus throughout your visit.

Think about some issue or concern or storyline you'd like more insight into. It might be a behavior or habit, your relationship with another person or group, or even a physical ailment. Phrase the question starting with "Give me insight into *[name your issue]*" and continue to hold your solar plexus chakra and breathe in through your nose and out through your mouth. Imagine the question sinking into the chakra, like water into soil.

You're going to travel downward, into your body, from where your hand sits on the surface. Imagine there's an underground parking garage below your hand. You're going to go down floor by floor to take soundings and gather insights. After you visit each floor, you will return to the surface, so you can take a moment to jot down whatever you heard, saw, felt, knew, tasted, smelled, understood, or thought there. If for some reason, you aren't comfortable with elevators, you can imagine another image such as stairs or ramps to get you from floor to floor.

Now, breathe in deeply, and imagine you are stepping into an elevator that will take you to each floor of the parking garage below you. Press the button for floor 1, the first floor down, and exhale, feeling yourself travel down the way you would in a real elevator. When the doors open on floor 1, step out into the space and tune in to what you encounter there. What do you notice particularly?

Keeping your original question in mind, ask the space, "What's your story?" Stay open to whatever comes to you in image, sound, knowing, or any form at all. . . .

Your first goal here is just to gather information, without judgment or trying to figure out what it means. Take your time to let yourself perceive what the space wants to bring to your attention.

If you sense something is needed, you are welcome to bring an antidote, do an energy medicine exercise while in that space, or call on the Universal Support Team to come help you out. But your main focus in this visit is to just let your understanding deepen and broaden in whatever way it can.

When you feel done taking soundings here, get back in the elevator, press G for ground floor, inhale through your nose, and feel the elevator returning to the surface as you exhale. Step out of the elevator. Take a few moments to jot down what you experienced on this first floor.

If you feel any reactivity to the travel, take a moment to do the Coming Home exercise: Place one hand on your solar plexus, the other on your heart, cross your ankles, and breathe in through your nose for a count of three, out your mouth for a count of five until you regain your equilibrium.

Ready to go to the next floor? Place your hand on your solar plexus, take a deep breath in, step into the elevator, press the button for floor 2, and as you exhale, feel yourself traveling downward to this new floor. Notice as you pass floor 1, perhaps as a friend you nod to in transit. And when the elevator doors open at floor 2, step out, and keeping your query in mind, ask, "What's your story?"

When you ask, take note of what arises, what you can perceive using all your senses. If you want to explore the space, you are free to do so, or just, if you wish, stay close to the elevator to take your sounding. If you find your mind wanting to rush to respond, intervene in what you're being shown, take another deep breath in through your nose and out through your mouth, and just listen and learn.

If you are feeling you have gotten your sounding, feel free to bring an antidote, do an energy medicine exercise, or call in guidance to help the energy you find there.

Then step back into the elevator, inhale deeply through your nose, press the button G for ground floor, and as you exhale, feel the elevator moving upward, back to the surface. Step out of the elevator and take a few moments to jot down what you've discovered there. If you find yourself reacting in any way, trace loving hearts on your heart or pet yourself behind the ears, like soothing a dog or cat.

When you are ready, inhale deeply through your nose, and step into the elevator, pressing 3 this time. As you exhale and travel downward, notice the floors you are passing, familiar spaces. Feel free to inhale and exhale as much as needed, letting yourself really feel you are traveling downward gradually to the next floor: 3.

When you arrive, keeping in mind your concern, ask, "What's your story?" Let yourself open to whatever you can notice. As before, explore the space as is comfortable. And if you wish to bring an antidote, do an energy medicine exercise, or call on guidance in this space, feel free to do so.

When you are ready, take a deep inhale through your nose, step into the elevator, press G, and as you exhale, feel the elevator rise back to ground level. . . . Jot down your observations without trying to nail down what they mean. If you need to calm yourself, do the Reconciliation exercise, holding your belly button and Mingmen area on your back behind your belly button, and let a figure eight travel between your two hands.

Now, if you're ready to travel down to floor 4, inhale deeply, step into the elevator, and press the button. Use your exhales to help power your descent to the fourth floor, letting the descent take time for your body to really feel the travel. Then step out, keeping your original search for insight in mind, and ask, "What's your story?" Take the sounding, tuning in to how the energy feels here, as well as what is calling your attention.

If you wish, bring an antidote, an energy exercise, or call on guides to join you here for a brief time. . . . And then when you are ready, return to the elevator, press G, and use your breath to power your rise to the surface.

Jot down your observations, calm your energy if needed, perhaps with a Consolation hold: right hand on your left ribs, left hand cradling your face.

And when ready, get in the elevator and press 5, remembering to breathe in through your nose and out through your mouth. And feel the elevator traveling deeper and deeper into your own being.

At the fifth floor, keeping your exploration topic in mind, ask, "What's your story?" and open all your senses to take a sounding where you find yourself. As before, if something needs to be addressed now, bring in gifts, an antidote, and/or helpers who can provide what is needed.

Step back into the elevator, push the G button, and use your breath to help you rise back to the ground floor. Feel the transit, and feel each floor you pass, places now more familiar to you. Once at the surface, exit the elevator and jot down whatever you noticed in your sounding. If you need to regroup, hold both knees, then both sides of your face.

When you are ready, it's time to go down to the sixth floor. Step into the elevator, press the 6 button, and allow yourself to feel the travel downward to this new level. Take your time, feel your breath moving in and out. At the sixth floor, step out, remember your intention, and ask, "What's your story?" Let whatever or whoever shows up inform you. Stay open to any storylines that pop into your head.

If you feel you want to, thank any folks you encounter at this level. Offer them gifts, or perhaps figure-eight them or between them and you. And when you are ready, return to the elevator, press G, and return to the surface.

Jot down details, and anything you noticed if you encountered others in this space. And if you need balance, place one middle finger in your belly button, your other middle finger at your third eye in a hook-up hold, and pull upward, breathing in through your nose and out through your mouth.

It's time for a visit to the bottom floor. Get in the elevator, press the button for 7, and feel yourself pass, one by one, the levels that are now more familiar. And at the seventh floor, get out, and open yourself to whatever you can perceive here. Do not worry if the energy or imagery feels different here. Just notice what you can. And, if you wish, invite your Councils or guides to join you in this space.

This floor is a great place to ask for a gift and give a gift, so if you want to, do that now . . . and then climb back into your elevator, press G, and use your breath to power your travel back to the surface.

Jot down what you experienced. Take a moment to read over all that you have written. Do not worry about making sense. Make sure you write down what the original request for insight was. Understanding might take some time to filter fully in.

Adjust your Acrobat's Pole front and back to make sure you are back in the *now*. Adjust your Torus Pole upward and downward to make sure you are back in your *here*. And spread your arms to adjust your Yin-Yang Pole, left and right, to find the balance point, then Celtic-weave across your chest three times, ending with both hands on your heart.

CHAKRA LEVELS AND DIMENSIONS OF SELF

As you review your notes over the next while to see what insights they give you, it can be helpful to have a general understanding of what dimensions of the self each level of the chakras roughly represents (going down in your elevator, starting with the first floor down):

Level 1: What is happening now in the *present story* of your life.

Level 2: What is relevant to the present *phase of your life* (the past month or two or three).

Level 3: What is relevant to the present *stage* of your life (the larger theme that may have been playing for several years).

Level 4: Who you understand yourself to be in this lifetime, based on the *identity* you have built through positive and negative experience.

Level 5: What *contracts or conditions* you set up to explore or express in this lifetime (including contracts to meet up and interact with others).

Level 6: What *past life or counterpart life events* are coloring your story (bleed-through from past lives).

Level 7: What *cosmic influences* are influencing your field (including bleed-through from other dimensions of reality and larger astrological tides).

● ● ●

When you are able to access your many dimensions, you can track your story-lines and get insights into how they express themselves and how they work, using the language of energy to renovate your creation of self.

In coming chapters, we will explore more ways to travel within the self and clear unwanted templates and storylines. We'll explore more Storymaker equipment, including what it uses to weave, source, and steer the ship. And we'll look at what this all means for healing and cultivating well-being.

CHAPTER SIX

Weaves of Meaning

Within the same week, I got called to help out in two extreme cases: both seventy-year-old women, ravaged by metastasized breast cancer, who were within a few days of dying. I suppose, given the era (it was in the late 1980s), some people only turned to energy healing as a last-ditch effort. On the other hand, I also recognized it as part of my Councils' curriculum.

In the first instance, a sweet elderly Asian man called me in to help his wife, Agathe, who was very ill, indeed. I saw at once that she was already beginning her transition out of this life. And she had made her peace with it: She was done. She was not fully conscious when I first arrived. All her energy was focused on taking the next breath, allowing her body to go through its process of separating, giving up the Radiance that had animated her for seventy years.

I sat quietly by her bedside, held her hand, and her husband left us together. In his mind, I was going to work a miracle. In my mind, her process of dying *was* a miracle. Despite her labored breathing, there was a deep sense of peace around her. She was not being killed off by the cancer; the cancer was her chosen exit strategy.

At one point, she opened her eyes, and skipping any preliminary chat, she said, with labored breaths, "There is nothing you can do . . . you know. . . . I'm on my way out. . . . Can you help him? . . . I agreed to have you come . . . to ease his mind."

"Yes," I said, "I will do what I can for him."

We sat like that for about an hour. I did some gentle energy communication to support her body to let go from the Web of Connections—to ease her systems, to support her choices. I could feel that her choices were not rooted in despair or failure to overcome the cancer: They were somehow coming from her soul's storyline. She had lived her life and this was her last page. As we just sat there together, she smiled, very deeply grounded within her being.

Finally, she squeezed my hand, indicating she was done with me. I asked her Councils to support her journey home and went to find her husband. I felt apprehensive, not knowing how to tell him there was nothing I could do to heal his wife and keep her in body. In fact, in her case, health was death.

I decided to just describe what I felt in her energies: Her deep sense of peace and completion. Her loving concern for him—how she wanted him to feel he had done a good job taking care of her. And that this was her choice: a successful exit from this life. And what I saw: that in the larger Web of Connections, they had a deep soul bond. And although her body was no longer viable, her soul and his were interwoven together.

As I heard these words coming out of my mouth, it surprised me a bit. I did not have a well-articulated spiritual belief system about life and death at that point. It was her Councils, guiding me in what to say, and his Councils helping him to hear the love and connection within the words.

He nodded and said, "I understand." It is hard to explain what was contained in those two words. He didn't have a shaktipat of awakening or take in my comments as concepts. He just felt, through the energies she and I had woven in that hour, that he was done too. I could see his need to save her draining out of him and a sense of peace and sad acceptance come in.

I didn't charge him for that visit. It was such a privilege to get that moment of sacred witness, to learn a bit more about the deeper connections forged by love and partnership.

So when I got a call later that week to ask if I could help another woman with advanced cancer, I remember thinking, *I've got this.* That should have tipped me off!

The scene I walked in on the next day could not have been more different. When the woman's partner, a young woman in her midthirties, met me at the door, she said, "Jodie is very committed to beating this cancer. She believes totally in energy healing and is excited you're here." The partner looked exhausted, drained, and freaked out. And when I walked into the room, where Jodie was lying in a hospital bed, stinking and visibly rotting as her body broke down, I could see why. Jodie was emanating energetic chaos. I've always thought of it as dog whistle energy: harsh, panicked, cacophony that maybe wasn't obvious to everyone, but it certainly grated on my tonal beagle ears!

Jodie was at least thirty-five years older than her partner, around the same age as Agathe, and though she was clearly in very bad shape, she was also clearly in charge of her own sickroom. She told me she *knew* she was very powerful, she had been a shaman in another life, and so when she got diagnosed with a cancerous lump, she had decided she would heal it on her own. She had read books and tried all kinds of visualization and had basically ordered the cancer repeatedly to leave her body, doing her best to impose her very impressive will on the situation.

"But I'm missing something," she said. "It hasn't responded, and I want you to show me how to get rid of this cancer."

The problem was that she had basically refused any treatment from practitioners (allopathic or alternative), shut out all helpers except her beleaguered partner, who she ordered around through my entire visit like an unsatisfactory servant. Clearly the partner was burned out. For good reason: The cancer had spread everywhere, and Jodie was just days away from death. Her body was basically saying, "She's not listening to me; she just bosses me around." Like the caregiver, Jodie's Gatekeeper was freaked out and burned out, and her Storymaker was stuck, like a broken record, on one story: She had to prove herself by vanquishing this disease.

Jodie's Councils said to me, "You can do what you can to try to help, but she has passed the point of no return. Unless she gets some emergency medical intervention, her body can't rally—and probably not even then."

Hmmm. I asked them to help me find the words and energy that might help Jodie and her partner. I have always been open to miracles and to healing that surpasses what my conscious mind might expect. But each time I tried to do something to help Jodie, she'd insist, "Tell me what you're doing. Tell me what is happening." And, energetically, she would pick apart the energies I was trying to help her Body Weave. (See page 156.) This was in between spasms of pain and difficulties breathing, because the cancer had already spread throughout her chest cavity and torso.

I did my best to explain what I saw going on. I affirmed her power, how strong her will was, but I also talked about how bodies don't like to be ordered about. "It isn't a matter of stronger willpower in this case," I tried to tell her in as uncritical a tone as possible. "It is a matter of finding the willingness to hear what your body needs."

In retrospect, I think Jodie knew she was dying. She seemed to be okay with that but not with losing face or being unable to use her psychic powers to heal her body. She had roped her partner into this determined effort to beat the odds, beat the cancer, beat the system, and was actually siphoning energy for her fight out of her partner (this was before the term "energy vampire" became vogue).

I told her honestly that her body was not responding to my efforts to communicate either. Her Gatekeeper had shut down and locked the doors. She had set up conditions that were impossible for it to work with. She not only had to heal with no medicines or interventions, but she also had to control the process as proof of her power. And her body and soul were saying, "Uh, no." Her body and mind were in a standoff.

I asked the partner to join Jodie and me, to sit and talk for a bit. I spoke for both of their Councils. And I talked about love—the partner's love in being willing to serve as a caregiver and Jodie's love of life demonstrated by wanting to vanquish the illness. But I pointed out how Jodie's choices were draining her partner's vitality and how her soul was asking her to learn to listen—to hear what her body needed and also to hear what her partner needed. It was asking her to change the terms of engagement. Her Councils appealed to Jodie's chivalry—I had a clear sense of some past lives for her as some kind of knight in armor or soldier. Could she release her partner to get some rest and call in some other helpers for a time? Could she allow a medical practitioner to assess where the cancer was at this phase, so they had better maps and insights into what they were dealing with?

I didn't need to tell her, "You are dying." They both knew it in their hearts. After about twenty minutes of discussion, Jodie said, in a quieter tone, "You know, I think I've already lost the fight. I can't fight any longer."

Her teachers said, "Then your path is to look at what you can embrace, moment by moment, where you find yourself. What your partner needs. What you need to do to clean up this mess."

Jodie and her partner thanked me for the insights, and again, I chose not to charge them (this time, because it didn't feel like sacred witness; it felt like an intervention!). The partner called me two days later to tell me that Jodie had contacted her doctor to get assessed, but then that same night died in her sleep. The partner sounded immensely relieved. She said, "I think she just needed permission to stop trying. Your visit did that for both of us."

ILLNESS, HEALTH, AND SOMETHING ELSE

Over the years, I have reflected back on these two women with the same diagnosis but very different situations who hit my radar the same week. Agathe had embraced her story's ending and was so ready to leave. She was doing her best to die with grace and in a way that supported her husband to let go. Jodie was exiting kicking and screaming, trying to impose a storyline and control the terms of engagement—to such an extent that she was draining her partner's life force trying to prove her power. I can imagine her soul, afterward, choosing another life where she could explore the differences between will and willingness! In this one, she had learned that her body could not sustain the storyline her will wanted to impose.

Although both were women around age seventy with terminal metastasized breast cancer, for Agathe the illness was her exit strategy: "Health" meant death, completing her journey. For Jodie, death was a wake-up call she heeded too late. "Health" would have meant confronting her need to control and prove her power. For her, the cancer (cells galloping out of control) lived a storyline that ultimately killed her. Both situations were not just about dying from cancer: They were about *what stories each woman had chosen to live.*

I have worked with lots of people over the years who were "healing into life and death," as authors and spiritual teachers Stephen and Ondrea Levine called it. Many with terminal diagnoses or diagnoses of *uncurable* chronic illnesses were able to learn a different style of partnership among their talking self, earth elemental self, and Wiser Self. And, in doing so, they were able to change the terms of engagement and bring in *miracle* healing.

Permission to find a different style of partnership with their bodies, for most of my clients, has always been a big part of the healing process. I've come to see it as a first step in healing (along with, of course, coming home to self). Allopathic medicine frequently addresses the symptoms of disease: What medicine will treat your high cholesterol, high blood pressure, cancer, migraines, pain, and the like? But energy medicine addresses what story you are living, what is needed for your story to evolve, and what you need in order to live well.

That does not mean you can't address the symptoms of high cholesterol in your body. It means that when you recognize the symptom as a flag, it tells you something about the energetics of your story and how you are living it. In response, you can shift the energetics and change the way your body is functioning.

It might be strange to say that we need permission to heal and permission to die, but our Western medicine, which suggests the doctor or medicine heals us, leaves many people believing (consciously or unconsciously) that both processes are out of our hands. Over the years, a good number of my clients came to see me in part to get permission to approach their healing differently: to look at possibilities beyond chemical or surgical interventions, to integrate their spirit into the healing process, to change the terms of engagement framing their illness, and to allow the possibility of healing their stories and their lives as well as their bodies.

In other words, I have come to believe that for many of us, part of healing requires us to rethink our beliefs about illness and health. If you are still reading this book, you probably believe that healing is, or should be, a whole-self activity, not just a body-based one. In fact, the root of the word "healing" is wholeness. But what does that look like in day-to-day life? How can we accomplish whole healing, particularly when we need to make decisions such as what to do about high cholesterol or blood pressure, aches and pains and hot flashes and emotional instability, hormonal imbalance, weight issues, and the like? In practical terms, most of us can't afford the sometimes-hit-or-miss process of finding alternative practitioners to help us think outside the box.

Rethinking Myths of Illness and Health

There is an art to being sick and getting well. First, we need to break the belief that sick is failure.

In our yes/no, right/wrong answer society, it is no wonder we tend to think in terms of being sick or being well. Something goes wrong, so we go to the doctor to get it diagnosed and fixed. We call that sick. And when the medication works and symptoms are under control, we tend to call that well.

But because we have been taught to think in such absolutist terms, we miss important understandings of both illness and wellness and the vast areas in between.

Agathe was dying of cancer, but she wasn't sick. She was breaking down at the cellular level as part of her exit strategy. Once her husband understood that, he was able to let her go, with love.

Jodie was in a battle of wills with her body. When she finally learned that her will could not control her body, she let go and died, far more peacefully than she had lived. In letting go, she also released her partner from unhealthy servitude.

Mindy, whose story I told in chapter 5, saw her multiple injuries and body pain as teachers inviting her to wake up, not as evidence of breakdown and failure. She used the exercises later in this chapter to reinstate her weaves of meaning that had gotten damaged in multiple car crashes and a traumatic childhood. And doing this freed her body, which had been bearing ongoing witness to the trauma, to repair itself.

The Purpose Versus the Meaning of Illness and Setbacks

I have a history of periodically coming down with an ailment my Councils called "Z flu." It was a flu with few specific symptoms: just exhaustion that sent me to bed to rest and sleep. The mild aches and pains acted as deterrents to keep me from moving around much. It was a recurring situation that would come up in certain circumstances:

1. When I needed to *prepare for something intense*, like helping someone birth a baby.

2. When I needed a time-out to let my energies adjust to some big *internal "rewiring"* process.

3. When I needed to *shift gears* emotionally, intellectually, and socially and might otherwise blunder along grinding my gears, rather than slowing down to push in the clutch, disengage, and shift.

When Z flu showed up, stopping in my tracks wasn't optional. It was the plat du jour. In chapter 1, I told the story of helping Sandra birth her baby. What I didn't mention was that within a few hours of telling Sandra I would help, I came down with a whopping case of Z flu. I spent three days in bed flat on my back feeling horrible, worrying that Sandra might call and I'd be too sick to help her. But on the fourth day, the day Sandra called me in, I woke up with batteries fully charged, ready to spend twenty-four-plus hours focused, channeling, and being the healer she needed me to be.

I later asked the Tibetans if they had any insight into Z flu and how to heal it. A number of them began to chuckle. In their cultures, they understood that a healer or shaman needed to conserve and gather power before a major "working." In those cultures, there was often a formula, such as "three days and three nights" of preparation, getting centered, consulting the Divine, and making oneself worthy to be an instrument of healing and vision. In our culture, doctors and even complementary healers tend to move from client to client, sometimes a new one every twenty to ninety minutes, with little preparation. It is just what is expected of us.

So how can we allow into our understanding of reality the fact that healing, for client and healer, may require more of us? My Councils used to ask someone who needed serious healing time, "On a scale of one to ten, where ten is overactive and one is pretty much comatose, where do you live your life?" Most of us live our lives at an average speed of seven or eight. They would explain, for repair of the body, healing speed is usually around three. Taking to bed *sick* and letting yourself hover at healing speed is not sickness; it is health.

Once I realized the purpose of Z flu, I was able to find ways to prepare for bigger workings without needing to feel like someone pulled my plug. I am mostly able, when Z flu shows up, to shift gears and put in my "three days and three nights" in greater comfort.

When you get sick or when unexpected events require you to reconsider your plans, ask yourself what purpose it is serving. Later, you can assess what it means.

Serving a purpose is different from asking, "What does it mean?" *Purpose* includes things like waking you up, giving you time out, flagging imbalance, slowing you down, showing you what processes aren't balanced in you, and allowing you to exit or undergo a death/rebirth. *Meaning* of an illness relates to what storyline you are living, what you are exploring as a soul. It relates to your weave of meaning and Web of Connections.

The purpose of Jodie's cancer was to force her to *wake up* to her skewed storyline about power or die. The meaning Jodie was exploring was the issue of will versus willingness. Her illness played that out.

Agathe's illness served the purpose of helping her husband let go of her, giving him time to adjust to her absence, like pulling off the Band-Aid slowly. Its meaning was a validation of their love and their vows to be there for each other in sickness and in health.

Think about the illnesses and so-called "failures" you have lived. What purpose did they serve? What meaning did they contribute to your life story?

I once got fired from a job I thought I loved. It was quite painful, emotionally and physically (I had frequent migraines and cold sores in response). My interpretation at the time was that there were jealous colleagues sabotaging my reputation. That was probably true. But putting myself in the victim seat was not productive, and in fact, it increased my suffering.

In retrospect, getting squeezed out of that organization was one of the best things that could have happened to me. At the time I worked there, I saw it as *the* path to the career I wanted. But, in the absence of that easy path, I had to bushwhack and create my own professional context. It acted like sand in the oyster. From that pain and hurt and sense of injury, I got pearls.

The *purpose* of the event was to create a death and rebirth in my life: to force me to let go of one storyline to get me to invest in another, better one.

The *meaning* of the event was that I was trying to get validation from a context that was not a good fit for me. It was part of a lifelong exploration for me of the theme of membership—what it means to belong, to fit in, to be part of a tribe.

> **Purpose** *relates to what your plot calls in to move you forward.*

> **Meaning** *relates to the themes you are exploring in this life as part of the storylines your consciousness and Storymaker are creating.*

You may not have a bigger picture when you are in the midst of the symptoms. On the other hand, if you can get some kind of framework other than "My body is falling apart; my health is failing; I took bad care of myself," you can harness the energy of what is happening and work with it. In many cases, that will reduce the physical pain and greatly reduce the mental suffering of finding yourself somehow out of commission.

Finding a productive framework that acknowledges your larger purpose, or what your soul is trying to achieve, or what the context has set for you as a challenge is crucial to healing. When we can see what is going on as productive, rather than merely as failure, we have more choice in how we respond and how we experience even the painful bits.

For example, when your infant has red, sore gums and is restive and screaming in pain, you most likely recognize your child is teething. With a reasonable framework, an explanation of what is happening and why, we don't generally rush our children to the hospital in a panic. We recognize that the pain relates to something good and productive: She's growing a tooth to help her chew. I call this kind of illness "emergence." With an illness of emergence, you might support the person in pain, but you aren't trying to stop the process. Food poisoning is similar: Clearing the stomach and digestive track is helpful, so you need to support the pain without impeding the process. That's an illness of "clearing," or "reset."

It is a myth in our culture that pain is bad: a sign of breakdown or failure or disaster or something wrong. Pain can also signal that your body or mind needs attention, adjustment, new dynamics, a change, or transition. Pain can usher in something better, more right. And like with childbirth, the opening can be uncomfortable, even if the result is something you may want. So it's worthwhile to explore what purpose your illness or setback or painful circumstance is serving, what life processes are influencing the health in your body and mind.

I've sorted some of the purposes I've seen over the years into four broad categories: awakening/activation, death and (re)birth, body on strike, and connection and membership. Play around with how these match your experiences of illness or setbacks.

Awakening/Activation

Ask yourself, "To what extent is this illness or event a *wake-up call . . . rewiring . . . shifting gears . . . course correction . . . refining the instrument . . . energy redistribution?*"

When someone is having a major spiritual, social, emotional, or intellectual awakening, they can get really dramatic symptoms: tumors, heart attacks, life-threatening acute illness, mental illness, digestive shutdown, and the like. Or they can just feel that they can't move forward or see to steer the ship. Your Gatekeeper does not like change, so the change implicit in awakening can trigger all kinds of symptoms and squawking on the part of your body and mind.

When I first started channeling, I said to a friend, "I think I'm having a nervous breakdown. I'm hearing voices." Luckily, she was wise and said, "You're not having a breakdown; you're having a psychic awakening!"

Death and (re)Birth

Ask yourself, "To what extent am I going through the stages of death and rebirth: *ending or leaving . . . loss/grief/mourning . . . gathering . . . gestation . . . time out . . . emergence/breakthrough . . . threshold sickness . . . energy redistribution . . . feeling new and vulnerable?*"

We go through many passages and phases in our lives, some shared with other people, some unique to our own personal path. And within those, we experience small deaths and rebirths repeatedly as we cycle along. When you can align with your phases, like aligning with the seasons, your Storymaker and Gatekeeper will be more comfortable with change, and your mind will navigate more comfortably.

Body on Strike

Ask yourself, "To what extent is my discomfort flagging that I'm losing the plot: *trying to live a storyline my body or soul can't accept . . . drainage or leaks in my energy circulation . . . infiltration or invasion of energies from outside . . . a need for different protection or to calm my Gatekeeper . . . too much or not enough energy in my protective shields . . . my well is empty . . . a need for energy redistribution . . . my body shut down for repair and reconstruction?"*

I have worked with many clients over the years who show up with pages of symptoms—and serial, chronic illness. A body on strike (either in shutdown or overdrive) serves the purpose of trying to get your attention in multiple ways. You've been giving it conflicting messages (or you've been absent), and your yin Gatekeeper (protecting your inner self) says, "I've got to shut you down." Your yang Gatekeeper (protecting you from the world) says, "You are pulling me this way and that way and you're in danger. And because that's happening, I won't go forward without better working conditions."

So rather than chasing the symptoms one by one or dealing with the multiple illnesses one by one, it's wise to renegotiate with the body on strike to figure out where there is positive motivation (for your talking self, your earth elemental self, and your Wiser Self) and reset your terms of engagement.

Connection and Membership

Ask yourself, "To what extent is this illness or breakdown flagging my disconnect from webs of connection (community, relationships): *templates of (past) trauma steering the ship . . . blockage rooted in fear or resistance . . . processing of sorrow, grief and loss . . . oversensitivity or lack of sensitivity . . . my sacred witness to some larger storylines of our shared humanity (such as when someone participates in a group disaster)?"*

We are designed to be part of webs of connection with others, and when those webs are either overpowering or distorting our own Storymakers or failing to give us the sense of connection we are wired to create, illnesses of body, mind, and spirit can arise. The energetics of connection and membership influence most of us more than we admit. Listen in to your internal monologue. How often are you calculating about what other people think, whether so-and-so's behavior is acceptable to you, or how to protect your reputation or be seen as your true self?

Take soundings, ask your Councils for guidance, and just give yourself permission to consider that illness isn't failure; it's part of the plot. This will help you begin to recognize what purpose your illness or dysfunction is serving, what it means in the context of your storyline, and how you can support yourself to shift the energy dynamics of your story that are keeping you from well-being.

WEAVING MEANING

Your Storymaker weaves energies into coherence to make meaning.

I am old enough to remember my mom when I was a kid, sock-darning egg in hand, manually repairing the holes in our socks. I loved to watch her carefully stitching along the edges to fill in and make the sock whole again. Well, mostly whole—they were usually pretty lumpy afterward. But the image of darning to make something whole again has stuck with me.

When something is off in your body, in your mind, in your story, it reflects that something is off in the weave of your subtle energies. Subtle energies, as I have said before, are not neutral. They each have a unique vibration that to a clairvoyant looks like color, to a clairaudient sounds like different musical tones, and to all of us encapsulate what we experience as *meaning.*

Merriam-Webster defines "meaning" as "the thing that is conveyed especially by language: import." In the language of energy, what has import is unique to each of us. It depends on your soul's purpose and spirit feeds, the conditions or contracts you set up to explore in this life, and the stories you have lived and experienced growing up. I find it fascinating to hear people talk about what they love: what objects, places, and activities have animated them and colored their story with meaning.

But when the basic weaves of our nature are torn, distorted, or destroyed in the course of living, our Storymakers find it difficult to create and hold on to meaning. Thus, healing your story and your Storymaker involves repairing and maintaining healthy weaves.

There are four weaves within our energy anatomy, in particular, that support us to live, love, and make meaning. And they are fruitful places to work energetically to heal from the inside out. I call these weaves the "Body Weave," the "Basket Weave," the "Web of Connections," and the "Safety Net." I'll explore the first three in this chapter and the Safety Net in chapter 7.

ⅢⅢⅢⅢⅢⅢ **Play with It!**ⅢⅢⅢⅢⅢⅢⅢ

This notion of having an underlying weave, a warp and weft, is powerful vocabulary in the language of energy. You can repair the weave and *darn* any part of your body where, like a worn sock, you feel the energies have lost their coherence and integrity. Repairing the weave supports the communications (probably via the fascia) that allow your body to bring healing resources to the area.

Find a place on your body where you suspect you need some repair to help support communication in the area or to repair something that isn't healing well.

With your finger, trace a circle or other shape around the area, to mark the edge you will be connecting up with your stitches. Then you have two choices:

1. You can use energy threads to graft a new weave over the area. Create a warp (vertical lines) and weft (horizontal lines weaving in and out of the verticals), and even, if you wish, use an imaginary shuttle to tighten the weave. Note: I often use long figure-eight motions to attach my threads.

2. You can make small stitches, as in darning, to fill in the space, working from one edge until you connect it up to the other.

In either case, feel free to choose colors and texture of thread that fit the situation. For example, you can use a favorite blue velvet thread, or threads made of forgiveness or clear thinking, or ask your Councils or the Universal Support Team to give you the most helpful threads to use.

After you are done weaving or darning, trace a five-pointed star and circle (see page 110) over the area to balance the newly installed energetic weave.

● ● ●

THE BODY WEAVE

Before I read any books or studied energy medicine, I was learning, apprentice fashion, through my hands-on practice, guided by my Councils and by individual healers from the World Wise Web group I came to know as the Tibetans. Because of this, my understanding of energy anatomy was not particularly systematic. And while I thought I was *seeing* energies, in fact, I was perceiving them with all my senses, often hearing, feeling, and knowing them rather than having a visual. When I did have a visual sense, it was often a metaphoric image, not the psychedelic lightshow true clairvoyants describe.

I had a lot of clients in my practice who were recovering from addiction, who had suffered trauma and abuse, and who were social outcasts. For example, even as early as the mid 1980s, I had a whole series of transgender strippers show up for healing work. And the energy feature that showed up for healing in many of these folks was what I called their "tennis racket."

Even before a client would tell me anything about their story, I could tell, from checking their tennis racket, whether they had experienced trauma. The tennis racket head was basically their torso area, and the handle extended down from their root toward (sometimes into) the earth. In people with trauma, there were broken strings, serious gaps in the crosshatch, cracks in the wooden head of the racket, and/or problems with the handle.

And I found that working to repair the racket made a big difference in how well they would heal and how well their Storymakers could create stories that allowed them to participate in playing the game of life. After all, if your racket isn't strung properly or isn't working, when you go to hit the ball, it makes a sick *thunk* and does not go where you intended.

Since that time, I've studied Donna Eden's fabulous grid-repair techniques and have come to call the tennis racket your Body Weave.* I perceive this weave as being something your soul lays down in creating you. The tennis racket I was seeing is the basic structure you build a self on in this dimension of reality. It allows you to set the strings to the proper tension to suit your circumstances.

In my book *Your Body Will Show You the Way*, I briefly introduced the Body Weave protocol to help reweave the tears in your fabric. I am bringing it back here as a crucial tool in repairing your Storymaker and offering some ways to deepen your understanding of how you can work with it to heal your story.

Protocol: Body Weave (with deepening practices)

1. Starting at the base of your left pelvis and at your left collarbone (the two points labeled 1 in Figure 6.1), hold your hands flat (or use fingertips if that is more comfortable) at the top and bottom to reinforce your first vertical warp line. It makes no difference which hand is holding the top or bottom of your Body Weave. Hold until you take a deep breath or feel these lines click into place and achieve a good tension (see Figure 6.2).

   If the line between these two points does not feel solid, you can reinforce it with color or sound until you sense it has a good, solid feel to it. Use whatever color or sound feels right. If this warp line feels like a clogged tube and needs clearing, blow downward sharply into (toward) the top as you would to clear a drinking straw or tube.

2. Move to the next two points on your pelvic floor and collarbone (the two points labeled 2 in Figure 6.1). Hold until you feel this vertical line click in or you take a deep breath. Adjust with color or sound and use breath to clear if needed.

---

* Donna Eden's Grid repair is an advanced technique requiring years of training and preparation on the part of the practitioner to handle the energies of doing it. I don't intend this Body Weave work as a substitute for Eden style grid repair but offer it as a self-help set of tools that complement that deeper work.

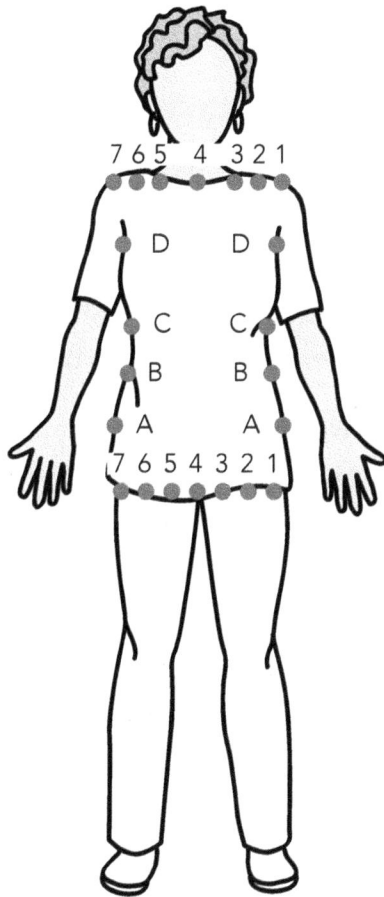

Figure 6.1.
Body Weave Points

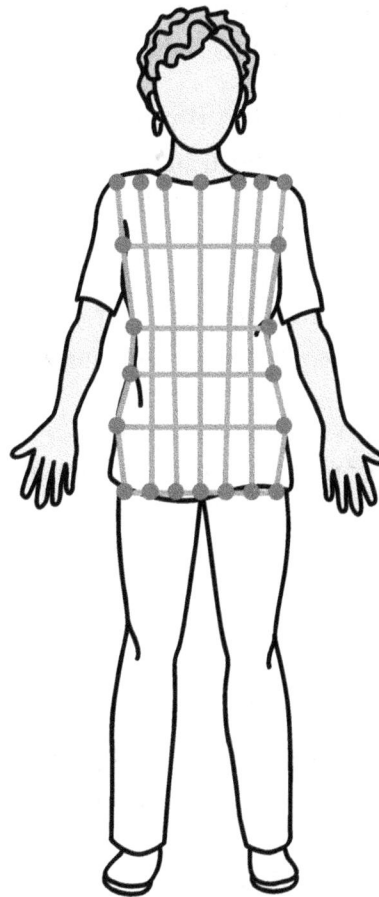

Figure 6.2.
Vertical and Horizontal Weave

3. Proceed to hold and reinforce lines 3 through 7 in the same manner, until you feel you have a solid warp to weave on.

4. Now it is time to weave your horizontal weft lines. Starting at the A point on your left side (see Figure 6.1), move your hand in a weaving in-and-out motion along your pelvic floor, as if you are weaving a horizontal thread over the first warp line, under the second, over the third, and so on. Continue until you have woven all the way to the A point on your right side (see Figure 6.2). Then hold the A points on the side

of each hip, both at the same time, until you feel this horizontal weft settle in and feel solid.

5. Continue to the B points at your waist. First use the weaving motion from left to right across your torso, and then hold both sides of your waist until you feel the weft line settle in and hook up.

6. Proceed to the C points at your rib cage. Again, make the weaving motion from left to right with your hand, and then hold both sides of your ribs until you feel the weft line settle in and hook up.

7. Next, weave in the same manner between your D points, and then hold and connect your D points at your armpits. You can hold with your thumbs tucked in your armpits and fingers covering the front of your shoulder, where your arm attaches to your body. Or cross your arms for this hold if that is easier.

8. Finish by tracing a figure eight on each of the diagonals, from left hip to right shoulder and from right hip to left shoulder. Then hold both hands on your heart, fingers interlaced, and breathe love and radiance into your renewed weave.

Deepening Practices

Going back to the tennis racket image for a moment, check the frame of your racket for cracks or nicks or anything that might affect its strength (see Figure 6.3 on the facing page). The head of your racket basically encompasses your shoulders, comes down along the sides of the rib cage, and then along your pelvic floor.

I still picture my racket as wooden, but you can play with whatever materials you wish yours to be. If there are cracks or nicks, ask the Universal Supply Team to give you energetic wood putty, superglue, or whatever is needed to repair it. Use gesture and touch to make these repairs, rather than doing it all in your head. Your body will know better what to do with the instructions when it participates in the repairs.

Then, check the handle of the racket. Is it intact? Needing repair? Needing the grip to be rewrapped at its base? Is it long enough to reach into the earth? Again, use gesture, and ask the Universal Supply Team for the necessary materials to bring it to its greatest integrity.

Because the Body Weave represents the energies laid down by your soul as a foundation in this life, just getting it re-established and rewoven is an important step. But since all energies have vibrations that your Storymaker uses in making meaning, you can tune in to each of the seven strings to ask, "What's your story?" This is a form of taking soundings at a deep part of your being. Often, you can get insights into what some of the terms of engagement are that were coded into your physical being to make it an instrument of expression.

Holding each strand, top and bottom (or left and right), take at least three deep breaths, in through your nose and out through your mouth, and ask, "What's your story?" or "Show me something about yourself." You can use the strands for divination as well, taking soundings: "Give me insight into . . . " You may find each has quite a story to tell!

Figure 6.3.
Tennis Racket Torso

Depending on your most comfortable processing type, you can interact further with your Body Weave in ways that make sense to your Storymaker.

1. If you are primarily *tonal*, you can interact with it as a stringed instrument. Tune each string using imaginary pegs at the top, letting your instinct guide you to know what tone each string needs in this moment. Then play this instrument. Let it amplify for you the music of your soul.

2. If you are primarily *visual*, treat your Body Weave as a tapestry. Bring a full rainbow of colored "threads" to allow you to embroider on the basic

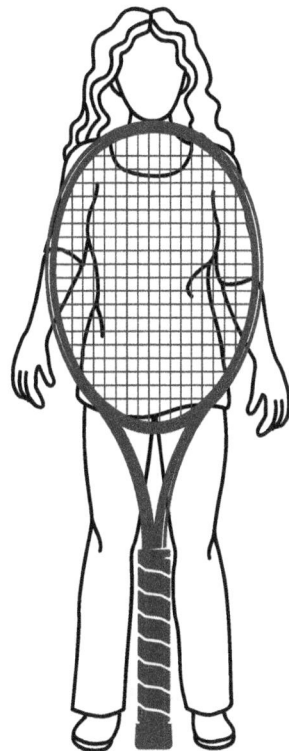

weave you've reinforced. What images and shapes want to emerge as you work with this canvas? What images or shapes are there that need to be picked out and replaced?

3. If you are primarily *kinesthetic*, once you have reinforced your Body Weave, place your hands in different parts of the weave and feel into it: What are you feeling? Use the feelings that arise as guides on what needs release, support, loving consolation, and augmentation.

4. If you are primarily *digital*, connect various parts of the weave with little hook-up holds (holding two points or body areas at the same time) while thinking about what you want to evolve in your story. Notice where the thoughts that arise are positive and productive and where they might be negative, judgmental, or perhaps not really logical. If you wish to offer reframes for these thoughts, do so, and then trace geometric shapes to bring harmony to the part of the weave where you are working.

BASKET WEAVE

One of the members of the Tibetan collective was a taciturn but clearly wise spirit who showed up in my practice with clients for several years to guide me. I called him the Old Chinese Gentleman, and I'm embarrassed to admit that I never asked his name or really sought to know much about him. What I did learn, over time, was that he was a Chinese shaman, who lived in the era when traditional Chinese medicine was being invented. He was big on five element (five phase) understandings but did not think much of the efforts to codify all the points and pathways so precisely. Not that I think we need get into age-old professional disputes!

Before I really knew what meridians were, he would point them out to me as *streams* of energy. He showed me various ways to work with them (mostly by diving into them and working from the inside), as appropriate for each client. I have since learned about meridians from my Eden Energy Medicine training and have a better understanding of how they are spoken of in healing literature. But, for the purposes of this discussion, let's call them streams.

Each stream brings a different *flavor* of energy, and to mix metaphors, I think of them almost as tones that together make up a scale or as crayons that together cover the color spectrum. On their own, the streams feed and support various organs. For example, spleen meridian feeds and supports the spleen and pancreas. Liver meridian brings energies to nourish the liver, and so forth. And so working with each of these streams can be very helpful in healing ailments in particular organs.

However, what is relevant here, in a discussion of weaves of meaning, is that there is a Web of Connections *between* and *among* the streams that underpins our energies. When one or more streams fall out of the weave, they cannot function efficiently and often drain the whole system. It is as if the meridians are all a collective that work together. The Basket Weave* represents this inter-relationship between meridians. When stress runs through the body's subtle energy systems, it disturbs the Basket Weave, leaving holes or disconnected relationships. And the weaknesses in your Basket Weave impede your Storymaker's ability to make meaning.

By repairing the Basket Weave, you are re-establishing harmony between meridian energies and stopping the seepage of energy (that is like bruising) from the system. Note: This is a great technique to help address general fatigue that is due to internal energy leakage.

When Mindy, survivor of seven car accidents, was connected in to herself enough to be able to communicate with her body's energies, she repaired her Basket Weave (page 165) to essentially clear the fog in her body's internal communications. Although she had no background in energy medicine, she just took one element a day, followed the instructions, and found that, within a week, not only had most of her pain lifted but also her bones, muscles, and tendons made a quantum leap in their recovery.

In Table 6.1, I list the elements (water, wood, fire, earth, and metal) with the names I learned to call the streams in my time with the Old Chinese Gentleman. Each element has two to four streams. The *flavor* of each stream

---

* Thanks to the fabulous Sara Allen for the name Basket Weave. The techniques I am teaching here are not related to the energy medicine she teaches about Basket Weave, but I have borrowed her phrase to refer to the interrelationships between meridians, as she does.

is named in the table (with the meridian name in parentheses). This will give you a sense of the energies that flow through our energetic wiring.

Table 6.1. Elements and Corresponding Energies

	WATER	WOOD	FIRE	EARTH	METAL
Conception (central)	Waters of Life (kidney)	Purpose (liver)	Heart Connection (heart) Yin Protector (circulation-sex)	Nourishment (spleen)	Give and Receive (lung)
Comprehension (governing)	Distribution (bladder)	Enactor/ Enforcer (gall bladder)	Choice/ Discernment (small intestine) Energizer (triple warmer)	Embodiment (stomach)	Distiller Refiner (large intestine)

If you, like Mindy, know nothing about energy medicine or five element theory, here's a quick explanation of the five-element (or five-pointed) star and circle. You've used it in a few of the earlier exercises in this book, tracing it to bring elemental balance. The glyph for this system is illustrated in Figure 6.5.

Don't be put off by how technical this looks! Each circle represents an element—water, wood, fire, earth, and metal. Within each circle, on the inner edge, you have initials for a *yin* stream: kidney, liver, heart, circulation-sex, spleen, and lung. And, within each circle, on the outer edge, you have initials for a *yang* stream: bladder, gall bladder, small intestine, triple warmer, stomach, and large intestine.

The star represents the inner balance between elements:

1. Water controls fire (because it can douse it).

2. Fire controls metal (because it can melt it).

3. Metal controls wood (because it can chop it).

4. Wood controls earth (because it can break it apart with its roots).

5. Earth controls water (because it can contain it).

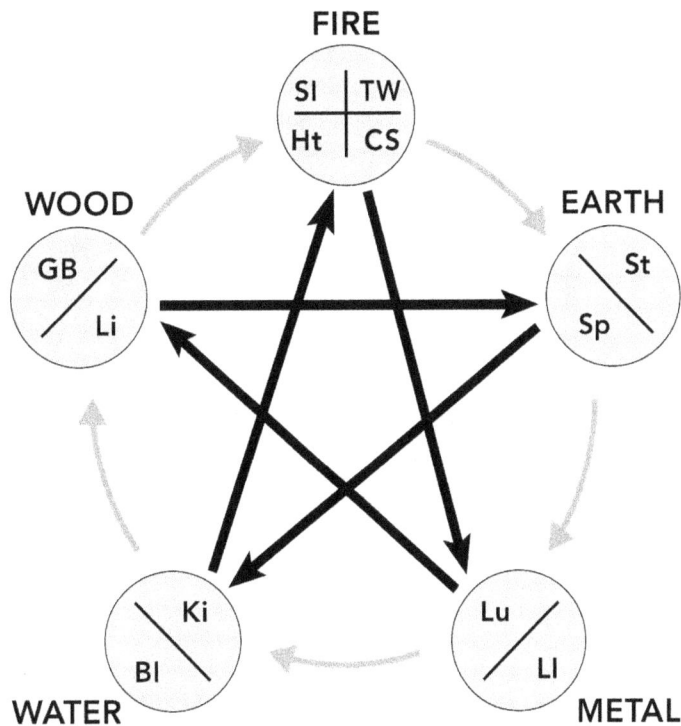

Figure 6.5.
The Five-Pointed Star
with Elements
(also known as the
Five-Element Star)

The circle represents the flow of elements, one into the other, usually starting with water.

To help Mindy remember this glyph, I gave her a thin glove with the image printed on it. If you wish, copy this page and cut the image out to glue to a glove or place on your hand!

Protocol: Basket Weave

To work with the Basket Weave, imagine the five-element wheel superimposed on the palm of your nondominant hand.* Fire sits at the base of the middle finger, water sits at the bottom lefthand corner, and metal sits at the bottom righthand corner (see Figure 6.6 on the next page).

---

* Thanks to Sarah J. Buck for her original creative insight that we can access the five elements via the hand.

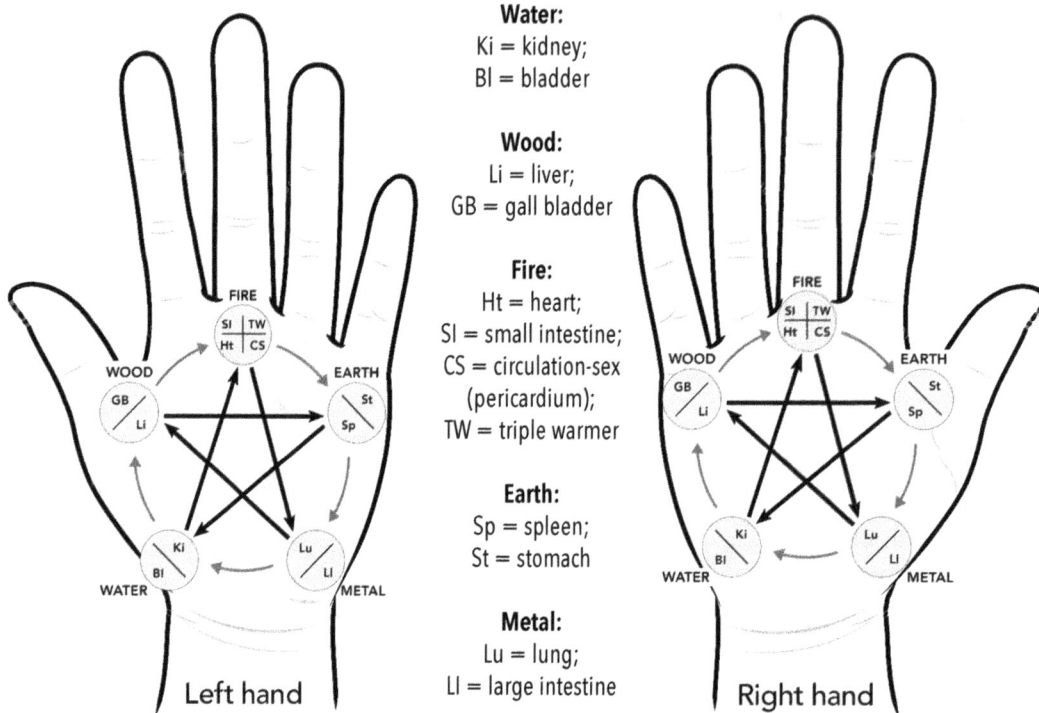

Water:
Ki = kidney;
Bl = bladder

Wood:
Li = liver;
GB = gall bladder

Fire:
Ht = heart;
SI = small intestine;
CS = circulation-sex
(pericardium);
TW = triple warmer

Earth:
Sp = spleen;
St = stomach

Metal:
Lu = lung;
LI = large intestine

Left hand

Right hand

Figure 6.6. Basket Weave on Palm of Nondominant Hand

The best way to reinforce or repair your Basket Weave, if you are just getting familiar with this five-element pattern, is to do what Mindy did, and do all five elements in turn, starting with whichever element you suspect needs it most. If you don't know, just start with water, and proceed to wood, fire, earth, and metal. You do not have to do all five elements at once. You might prefer to do an element a day over five days and tune in to what it affects.

1. Start with a single *yin* stream or focus meridian. For example, if you start with water, you'll touch on your hand where you see Ki (kidney).

2. Trace figure eights on your hand between the focus meridian and its yang partner (like in square dance, do-si-do the partner). In the example, you would figure-eight between Ki (kidney) and Bl (bladder).

3. If the focus meridian is a *yin* meridian, now figure-eight between the focus meridian and each yin meridian on the wheel in turn. In the example of kidney, you would figure-eight kidney + liver, kidney + heart, kidney + circulation-sex (pericardium), kidney + spleen, kidney + lung.

4. Then again figure-eight between the yin and yang (do-si-do the partner). In the example, figure-eight between kidney and bladder.

5. Then figure-eight between the focus meridian and each yang meridian in turn. For example, kidney + gall bladder, kidney + small intestine, kidney + triple warmer, kidney + stomach, kidney + large intestine.

6. End by do-si-do-ing the partners once again. In the example, kidney + bladder.

This brings your target meridian (stream) back into the Basket Weave and repairs the interconnections. Once you have completed the yin partner, it is good to Basket Weave the yang partner in the same session.

If the focus meridian is a *yang* meridian, follow the same pattern, but link first with each yang and then with each yin (here's what it would look like for bladder meridian):

1. Do-si-do between bladder and kidney.

2. Figure-eight between bladder + gall bladder, then bladder + small intestine, then bladder + triple warmer, then bladder + stomach, then bladder + large intestine.

3. Do-si-do once again between bladder and kidney

4. Then figure-eight between your target (bladder) and all the yins: bladder + liver, bladder + heart, bladder + circulation-sex (pericardium), bladder + spleen, bladder + lung.

5. End by do-si-doing the partners: bladder + kidney.

If you use the diagram in Figure 6.6, you can just follow the pattern without needing to worry about the names of the meridians.

It is possible to work with just the individual elements or streams that have fallen out of the Basket Weave. You can either touch each position and feel into whether it is secure in the Basket Weave.* Or if a particular issue is up for you, start with the meridian that makes logical sense. For example, if you're having problems with digestion, start with the earth element. Or if you are having trouble with emotional flare-ups, start with fire.

THE WEB OF CONNECTIONS

My image for the Web of Connections is like a neural network: a weave of energies wired together to create meaning. But the Web of Connections is not within our brains. It is our energetic interconnectedness with all sentient beings and with all Consciousness. Just as you can get information and influence from the World Wide Web when you tune in to it and search, you can get energetic feed and guidance from the collective of beings and from other individuals via the Web of Connections.

That's the positive aspect, like the convenience of googling to get information at your fingertips. The negative aspect is one that many of us have been experiencing for some time, perhaps since the invention of the internet. It is the fact that we are influenced and swayed by energies coming at us: by other people's values, stories, actions, noise, and efforts to claim power. In that sense, life on this planet is not a solo journey; it is a collaborative effort, and we don't usually have much control over who we are collaborating with.

I am reminded of those treasure hunts where a group of people is jointly charged to find the treasure, and each member is given a handicap, so they have to work together and cooperate to get to the goal. Life sometimes feels like that. It is both painful to have to accommodate different agendas and rewarding when we manage to move the group forward.

---

* If you are familiar with energy testing, you can also energy test while touching the target (or touching the target together with another stream). A weak test shows an element that has fallen out of the basket. This is a more advanced application for those of you using these methods with clients.

But though the Web of Connections, like the internet, is vast and filled with influences you as an individual don't want, it is manageable when you learn how to call in what you choose, to filter out what is not in alignment with your purpose, and to form tribes of affiliation that, like the neural networks, favor the positive connections over those that don't feed you or fit your soul's purpose.

I think of this as forming your own World Wise Web—your network of supports, kindred spirits, tribe, and affiliations that, by their nature, strengthen your ability to access wisdom that fits your soul's truth and help you filter out the irrelevant *noise.*

Although I have been blessed to build relationships with my Councils and further, to find my affiliations as a healer through joining the Tibetans group, this is not unique. Whether or not you recognize it, in addition to the communities you have consciously joined, you have membership in your Councils (hopefully you've been able to start getting to know them) and you belong to inner/outer groups through your Wiser Self. It is likely you have contact with these kindred spirits while you are sleeping, in moments of revery, when you are meditating or swimming or showering or walking or making art, letting your imagination run wild, recognizing something familiar in someone you have just met, or in other activities that open your mind to high-quality energies.

Like with the internet, the first aspect of working with the Web of Connections is to recognize how you let the energies in and establish filters that bring in only what serves you. In other words, it is good to create your own "algorithms" to help you make the connections with other people and influences that support your mind-body-spirit journey in this life.

On page 58, I mentioned the Smart Filter—a simple energy exercise that involves figure-eighting the edge of your aura to help it do a better job of filtering what can come into your field from the Web of Connections. So that's a place to start. And then I believe in putting out invitations, calls to our kindred spirits inviting them in. By kindred spirits, I don't just mean the woo-woo kind—you may or may not be comfortable inviting them in. I mean those people who just resonate with you for some reason.

Start collecting symbols of what you would like to call into your life. You may already know someone who speaks to something deep in you. Use a picture of them (to say to the Universe, "Send me more like this, please!"). You may feel drawn to essences such as objects from nature that stir something in you. You may have words or talismans or cards from a divination tool that seem to capture something of what you'd like to call in.

Place these objects in a circle around you, at a little more than arm's distance from your body. Then figure-eight between you and the Web of Connections, the world around you, with these objects at the center of the figure eights. Imagine them growing, becoming part of a filter that calls in the energies they represent and protects you from energies that won't serve you.

If you have met your Councils or any guides you trust, invite them to join the circle around you, and ask them to help you send out requests via the Web of Connections, calling in your kindred spirits, calling in energies that will nourish and feed your purpose. If you want to play with sound or color, you can sound different notes that seem relevant or bathe the invitations in a color that speaks to you in this moment.

When you have finished, thank your guides, collect your talismans, and put them each somewhere in your house to help continue to call in the energies you are inviting into your World Wise Web.

● ● ●

The more you can support your weaves, the more your Storymaker will be able to create a meaningful story in alignment with your Wiser Self. The other night I was feeling unraveled and unable to even call to mind all these great techniques for repairing my weave. I was in bed, tired, fighting some kind of bug, and too lazy to deal with it.

My Councils suggested I wrap myself in a "story blanket." They said, "Ask your Wiser Self for a blanket, imprinted with your best stories, your greatest truth. And wrap it around yourself, all tight and cozy. Let the weave of the blanket, the stories woven into it, seep into your very fibers. Let the Universe restore you to wholeness."

It was a good reminder that, sometimes, we also need to just let go and let ourselves be helped!

CHAPTER SEVEN

Sourcing and Steering

When my friend told me I was having a spiritual awakening, not a nervous breakdown, she said, "Go get a book by Alice Bailey." I knew Alice was an old-timey metaphysical author, so the next day, I headed out to a New Age bookstore I'd seen in passing. As I walked along the street, feeling expansive, happy, and a little keyed up, I thought, *I need a job one day a week.* I was a student at the time. I walked into the bookstore and found Alice Bailey's books, which were all in identical unadorned blue covers. I chose the one that seemed to be first in the series and took it to the counter. The man behind the counter, a kind of distracted, sleepy-looking guy, looked up and said, "You wouldn't be interested in a job one day a week, would you?"

A few years later (perhaps the early 1980s), that encounter and silly little job and a visiting speaker who canceled brought me into a group of people who were all spiritual seekers. There were about nine of us disappointed that the speaker was a no-show, so we went out for snacks. We decided to start meeting regularly to compare our experiences with "awakening." It was a diverse group: We had a couple of Fam-Trad witches (initiated and trained in a tradition handed down from one generation to the next), a few astrologers who were also old-timey kabbalah-style occultists (pathworkers), a woman who had a deep practice as a Quaker, a few shamans, and me, who by that point had been in training with my Councils several hours each day for a couple of years, trying to understand who these new inner teachers I'd let into my life and mind were.

It was a fascinating process, sharing notes about how each of us perceived various topics in consciousness. *What does your tradition say? What practices do you do?* What amazed me most about that group was the sense of how we had all arrived at very similar kinds of awareness by wildly different paths.

During those early days of awakening (and maybe ever since), the world seemed to shine with meaning. Small moments took on symbolic significance, and over and over again, I'd have these weird coincidences of thought and reality coming together like that. It wasn't just little psychic hits (though those have continued). It was as if the ingredients would all line up so I could bake the cake I needed to bake, without my needing to pull them off the shelves or put together my shopping list. I mean that metaphorically, of course. My life felt guided—in a light but extremely helpful way.

The Alice Bailey book was a bit of a bust, though. I plowed through what seemed like impenetrable prose and word sludge until I got to the part where she said, "If you can't understand what I am saying, you aren't ready to know it." *Well! Okay, then,* I thought. *I guess I'm not ready to know it.* I owned all the Alice Bailey books eventually, one of the perks of my bookstore job, and ended up carting them through one move after another, though I never did get enough enlightenment (or patience) to swim in those waters.

Not only are there many paths to awakening, but also from what I can tell, some of them involve slogging through some pretty thick concept-soup. I remember one day many years later (maybe the twenty-teens), when I was working as a conscious channel, doing readings and spiritual coaching. I had a client who had come from a weekend workshop and was beating herself up for not being able to activate her "Merkaba." This was new to me at that time. According to Google:

> *Merkaba,* also spelled *Merkabah,* comes from a Hebrew word meaning chariot, or vehicle, and can also be defined also as light, spirit, body. The Merkaba Symbol is a shape made of 2 intersecting tetrahedrons that spin in opposite directions, creating a 3-dimensional energy field. . . . The merkaba is said to provide protection and transport your consciousness to higher dimensions. The merkaba shape reminds us of the potential power we can wield when we unite our own energies in pursuit of connection and growth.*

---

* Soul Flower: Finding Soul, "Merkaba Symbol – Sacred Geometry," November 16,

It is an interesting concept, but we had to spend most of the session exploring why she would beat herself up with how she *should* be awakening and how inadequate her lack of Merkaba made her feel. In those days, I met so many people getting inspired by New Age theories and beliefs and then applying them to their lives as something they needed to accomplish or measure up to.

Another woman, that same day, announced to me that she had achieved "fifth dimension consciousness" and intended to live until she was 140 (you can google that one yourself!). She was seventy at the time. And I felt embarrassed. I had read a book about the fifth dimension sometime in the eighties, but it had gone in one head and out the other. What was this 5D she assumed I should know? Here's the thing: She may indeed have achieved this state of consciousness, but it was clear to me her path was seriously blocked. In fact, the next day, she was diagnosed with a return of breast cancer, stage 4 and metastasized. Far from living to 140, she was actively dying.

There might be something to this fifth dimension stuff though, because she walked an inspiring path to death in a way that brought light to the people who loved her. But sometimes there is a significant distance between our *belief* about consciousness gleaned from books or online courses, and what our lived experience looks like.

I often think we are in an era of change similar to the times of Christ and Buddha, when teachers and messiahs abounded, when people were awakening but also falling into weird and extreme practices and using their beliefs to try to control others. In our time, we have hordes of people striving to awaken, to evolve their consciousness, and other hordes fighting it, ironically using the term "woke" as a pejorative. (Though what is the positive value there—asleep at the wheel?) And for both groups, we now have the multiplying factor of the internet, amplifying the beliefs and groupthink, using spiritual memes or anti-awakening tropes to get buy-in and followers in ways that are probably not conducive to personal grounded enlightenment.

When we say we are awakening, what are we awakening to? Personally,

---

2018, https://www.soul-flower.com. https://www.soul-flower.com/blog/merkaba-symbol-sacred-geometry/#:~:text=Merkaba%2C%20also%20spelled%20Merkabah%2C%20comes, a%203%2Ddimensional%20energy%20field.

I don't think it's about quantum physics or new kinds of spiritual-scientific understandings of *reality* (though they are interesting, for sure). I don't even think it's about taking on superpowers, though I find that one more tempting. My partner knew a woman in the 1970s who could turn on light switches with her consciousness. For some reason that stuck in my mind as something I would love to be able to do. But when I take a moment to reflect, I have to admit it's a rather random goal since we have remotes that accomplish the same thing.

I think garden-variety awakening includes a number of things: presence, a greater fluency in the language of energy, and the ability to see things from many perspectives, with compassion . . . for starters. Ruth Denison, a crusty old German Buddhist meditation teacher I sat with for many years, was incredibly psychic. It had opened in her naturally as part of her awakening and enlightenment. I remember her saying (in her thick German accent), "Forget all that psychic stuff; it's a lot of distraction. Bells and whistles. Do you KNOW you are breathing?"

Enlightenment means turning the light on inside you, which helps you see the light in all of life. It is not an idea or explanation of reality. It is the ability to actually tune in and discern the many levels of reality, and the wisdom, as they say in AA, to "know the difference" between what it means to inhabit your truth versus just speaking knowingly about someone else's.

This is the realm of your Storymaker: the place where your truth gets assembled and formed. Your Storymaker helps frame and codify your beliefs on many levels:

- The beliefs about reality you've internalized

- The myths you were told about yourself

- The stories you tell about yourself

- The beliefs you carry about yourself*

---

* Shoutout to DeeAnn Weir Morency, Unity Minister and coauthor of *Discover Your Divinity*, whose PowerPoint slide in a recent talk inspired this list.

Beliefs are more than thoughts in your head. They form the inner architecture your Storymaker relies on to interpret experience and reality. And, as such, we need to be able to work with them, not just as thoughts but as energy structures.

To me it comes down to this: What beliefs help you get nourished and bring you home to your inner truth? And what beliefs block you, tie you in knots, disempower you, or keep you *out there* in realms of abstract thought and understanding, divorced from your own experience and knowing?

|||||||||||||| **Play with It!** ||||||||||||||

What are you personally being asked to awaken to? Try this multi-dimensional self-interview process. Ask yourself the questions listed here, one at a time, perhaps even one a day, to hear your own path communicate to you.

Rather than just plumbing what your brain thinks about it, take *soundings* of your whole mind—at different places in your body that seem relevant to you. Let yourself get insights in many forms: imagery, feelings and sensations, sounds/words, rhythms, direct knowing, movement, gesture, abstract shapes, or colors.

Gather those insights together, and then see if your mind can find language to name what you perceive, using metaphors, made-up words, or whatever can get you past the vocabulary your trained brain is expecting to apply. You might even want to assign a name like Gertrude, and then describe who Gertrude is, as an important character in your life story.

1. What do I know about my inner truth?

2. How can I most readily access my inner guidance?

3. What do I know about my inner affiliations?

4. What is my creative nature? In what ways am I a creator?

5. What are my sources of anchoring and security and connection, both in my life and within myself?

6. How much love do I feel for life, the world, this human experiment?

7. What limits and blinders enable me or block me from exchanges with the world at times?

8. How does my yearning to come home to my truth express itself in my life and choices?

9. How do I express or act on my yearning to connect to the world?

10. What is my guiding story right now about myself and about the world?

11. To what extent is my mind coming up with stories, interpretations of events, that thwart my evolution or don't allow me to change?

12. What larger patterns and mission have I signed on for?

13. What contracts, implicit or explicit, frame my choices (and limit or empower me)?

14. What is my relationship to change—in practical terms and in the landscape of beliefs and ideas?

15. What roles do I play in the collective weave? What do I bring to the shared fabric of our collective cultures?

16. To what extent do I feel free to select from the collective weave those threads that fit the patterns I wish to be living?

These are big questions that you don't need to find definitive answers to. They are worth returning to periodically, since even asking them helps you open the drawstring bags of your mind to allow new life in.

Whenever you find yourself reading an author or listening to a presentation where someone is explaining the nature of reality to you, defining the inner realms using science or even configurations gleaned from age-old spiritual traditions, remember this: Your Storymaker can learn from these, but to stay healthy and serve you, it needs *you* to be the author, creating your own explanations, co-creating truth that makes sense from the inside out.

SOURCING

"On paper," Dorothy said, "I just had my perfect year. As a gift to myself for turning forty-five, I lost fifty pounds, which was my heart's dearest desire. And then I got a promotion at work, into more of a leadership position, again something I'd been wanting for some time. And my team created an amazing app, which I'm going to get royalties from. But I am numb. Instead of feeling happy and fulfilled, I'm feeling lost and disoriented, at best, and often I just feel nothing. I've been trying to hide this from myself and also from all the people who come up to congratulate me on my new looks and new position. What can I say? It wasn't nothing. But it sure doesn't feel like I thought it would!"

The energy dynamics in Dorothy's story all pointed to a dysregulated Storymaker, in particular its ability to *source* her and her ability to *steer* the ship and to navigate life confidently as a result.

> *Sourcing relates to how you get nourished. Where do you get fed, inspired, taught, both from within and outside yourself? What is your equipment for access to nourishment and how can you repair and maintain it?*
>
> *Steering is the capacity your Storymaker has to steer you in life, to give you a sense of direction, orientation, and destination.*

We dove a little deeper into Dorothy's story. She had lost her weight using a popular online program that combined psychological insights with learning healthy eating habits. She sounded defensive: "It wasn't some crazy crash diet or anything!" What she learned in the process was how she had repeatedly used food to soothe herself and to insulate herself when she felt others were making demands on her. She had carried around the extra fifty pounds as a ready excuse: If she failed, she could blame her weight and other people's prejudices. If she succeeded, she could be a hero, overcoming the stereotype to prove her worth.

"I learned I have to always eat in quiet surroundings," she said. "If other people are stressed around me, I just take in their stress, and it interferes with my ability to know when I've had enough. And the program had us look back at what we learned about food and eating as kids. My mom was a very anxious person, and an overeater herself. What I remember was that she would offer food whenever we were sad, or hurt, or angry about something." She went on, "My problem is that all these insights helped me succeed in the program and lose the weight, but then I got busy at work, so it has taken most of my time and attention to just stick with the new eating habits and not regain the weight. I'm still a fat person inside, and to be honest, I feel somehow broken in there most of the time."

Dorothy had discovered two things. The first was that her imbalanced relationship with food had kept her from learning how to cultivate nourishment, fulfillment beyond what she could get from food (like with alcoholics, missing out on what they might have been experiencing). And, second, she learned that below the emotional, psychological story is often an energy story and some equipment that is broken or not working properly. Like Dorothy, it is useful to ask, "How well is my Storymaker functioning? How did it learn to make stories, to frame my experience, and to give my life meaning?"

For whatever reason, Dorothy's mother had not known much about how to nourish her daughter beyond the obvious: feeding her. And since food includes not only sustenance but also stimulants and numbing agents, Dorothy had used feed-and-pacify patterns to meet her needs. And she had often used sugar to bring the sweetness that would lift her above that dull feeling deep down.

What jumped out at me in Dorothy's story was a disconnect between inner and outer for her. It is the Storymaker's job to codify and integrate inner and outer experience to create your Safety Net, to frame your lived experience. It enables you to participate in the larger Web of Connections, in part based on how well you learned to get nourished within and from your environment.

Dorothy had a lot going for her in her life: She was competent in her work, and her body was reasonably healthy. But this disconnect between *getting* the things she wanted and being able to actually *have them*, take them in, be nourished by them, was making her feel she had lost the plot of her life. What do you steer toward if getting there doesn't really feel like much? Dorothy was reasonably savvy about the psychology of what she was living. But she had not yet activated or repaired the energy systems that gave rise to her feelings (and lack thereof).

Our work together focused on helping Dorothy get to know and use her Storymaker equipment, particularly her Umbilical Passage, Mingmen Passage, and Safety Net. She also had to learn to adjust her energetic steering mechanisms to allow her to do more than just set goals and reach them.

The Umbilical Passage

When we are in our mother's womb, we are sourced via our umbilical cord, through which we get both oxygen and nutrients. Equally, we are sourced by our mother's womb and body, creating a field of literal and energetic supports to our evolution. Then we are born, the cord is cut, and we have to learn to get our needs met from the world and people around us.

For some of us, learning to breathe, learning about the world, getting to experience first being fed and nurtured with breast milk, and later learning how to take in and digest foods from the earth is an enjoyable process. We are fed by love and care, nourished by exploration of the world and people who teach us, by sound and language, by visual stimulation, by action and interaction, by getting to know our earth elemental self, and by objects we interact with to form experiential understandings of what this dimension of reality is all about.

If any of that process was fraught for you as it was for many of us, you probably have built stress, tension, distrust, pain, fear, and hunger into your Storymaker's sense of self and world. It keeps your Gatekeeper on alert, protecting you from conditions that may or may not still be present. So claiming your ability to be nourished includes evolving your instrument to make and live story differently.

Umbilical Passage is the name I've given to the energy feed that you can access via your belly button. Just as amputees can often feel their missing limbs because their energy body still retains the energetic limb, we still have an energetic umbilicus: an energy cord we can use to get nourished, even when the world around us seems pretty toxic.

Your Umbilical Passage starts at your belly button area and extends outward from there as a hollow cord (basically similar to our literal umbilicus when we were in the womb). The problem is, for most of us, ignorant that our energetic feed is still there once our flesh cord was cut and tied, it just flaps in the wind—randomly serving us or not, or worse, taking in toxins unknowingly because our Gatekeepers don't realize they are supposed to be protecting us there. Here is a guided visit to help you get to know—and heal—your Umbilical Passage.

Guided Visit: Getting to Know Your Umbilical Passage

Like with all guided visits, it is important to make sure you are in a safe and comfortable place, with time to explore and let the experience unfold for you. Do whatever preliminary breathing and centering activity you need in order to be present for yourself. See page 13 for instructions on how to access the MP3s.

Take a moment to feel the area of your belly button. . . . Wrap your hands along the energy tube extending out from that area to feel into it. What can you perceive about it? Is it calm and happy? Nervous and stressed? As if it were a preverbal infant, hold the tube, embrace it and console it, bring it into communion, as a loving mother does for her newly emerged baby, trying to make her infant feel the same love and protection it had in the womb.

Breathe in through your nose, and exhale oxygen and nourishment through your hands, infusing your energetic umbilical cord with whatever you sense it most needs right now. Continue this until you feel a shift in the energy, a *coming home* for your Umbilical Passage.

Then, move your hands outward along the umbilical tube, to the portion beyond where you were just holding. Again, tune in to the energy of it. Embrace and console it. Bring it into communion with your own loving heart.

Continue this process outward along your Umbilical Passage. Discover how far out it extends or wants to extend, and keep meeting and bringing the energy into your understanding of yourself. This is a sacred part of your energies you may not have recognized since you were in the womb. Or perhaps you have recognized it, so you can use this time to clean it of whatever energies have slimed it in your efforts to get nourished and breathe in this world. You can use whatever comes to mind to clean it—wiping it with a soft cloth, using a stream of warm water, bathing it in light or sound, asking the Universal Support Team to come in to help.

Now, find someplace you feel you can trust to anchor your energetic umbilical cord, hooking into a source of nourishment. It might be a place that speaks to your deepest nature, it might be the heart of the Divine, or it might be a place you imagine such as the "well of restoration." For now, it is probably best to choose something bigger than yourself (e.g., a mountain, a tree, a Divine being) rather than another person.

Now, return your hands to your belly button area, forming a heart shape around your belly button with your two hands (as you see many in popular culture doing to signal love to a crowd). Breathe in through your nose, and send love out through your hands, with the exhale, into your Umbilical Passage. Then inhale, and as you exhale, sink your consciousness down into your belly area, to the inside of your belly button, to the place in your belly underneath the knot. Use your fingers to gently mime untying the knot to open your Umbilical Passage up again. Take your time with this: If the knot is tight and old, you might need to ask for help from the Universal Support Team, or ask for some energetic salve to soften the tissue and allow it to open.

If you are nervous about unwanted energies entering or exiting your newly opened entrance, put an automatic screen and door there, coded to only allow energies for your highest good to enter, coded to only allow energies that are in support of your truest nourishment to travel this conduit.

Take a deep breath in and then exhale, feeling your way into your Umbilical Passage. Tune in to what you can perceive there: Is it healthy and vital, or does it need some repair? Maybe the walls got damaged and need to be patched up. Maybe the tissue is tough and full of scars. Call out through the World Wise Web for a healer who is expert in umbilical repair, in restoring your Umbilical Passage, and invite them in to help you reclaim and rehabilitate this important energy passage.

Travel in through the passage, assessing what is needed, getting help with repairs and replacements as needed. This can take some time or even several visits, or it may happen spontaneously for you, depending on what stories your Umbilical Passage has lived in this and other lives. Remember, you can always repeat this visit if this part of your energy anatomy needs some taming, like a neglected dog who has not yet learned to trust.

Keep breathing in through your nose and out into the Umbilical Passage, using your breath to clear detritus and help it open.

When you are finished with this present visit, return your attention to your hands, cupping your belly button in a heart shape. Feel your energetic umbilical cord, noticing whatever you can about how it has shifted during your visit. Know that the work you did can continue; the repairs can sink in and be assimilated. Thank any helpers you brought with you do this work.

Now reach out and unhook your Umbilical Passage from wherever you anchored it, wrap it around and around your body, in a spiral, encasing your body, and hook it into your heart as a place to rest.

· · ·

Your Umbilical Passage is a magical and mysterious energy feature. As you get to know it, it can reveal its capacities to source you, to seek and bring in nourishment. Whenever you are not sure where your nourishment is to be found, whether a situation is healthy or destabilizing, you can unhook your Umbilical Passage from its resting place in your heart and send it out as a feeler and guide to help you discern what will nourish you.

You can use it as a cord, when appropriate, to plug temporarily into a source of inspiration you trust to help you bring that inspiration in deep to nourish you. But like a plug-in car, be conscious that you don't want to try to drive off while plugged into something outside yourself!

Since we live in a time of demagogues and cults, I suggest *not* plugging into people, no matter how inspirational they are or how much you love them. Just as we are meant to exit the womb and individuate from our mothers, it is not necessarily a healthy choice to try to make someone else your mother or some outside situation your new womb. Sourcing, once we are out of the womb, means accessing oxygen, water, food, and energetic resources from the world and processing them through our literal and metaphoric digestive systems. The Umbilical Passage then becomes a conduit for nourishing connection with the world around us.

Dorothy used her Umbilical Passage as something like a combination of a vacuum cleaner and an elephant's trunk. She would send it out to pick up information she suspected was out there that she couldn't quite perceive, and suck it deep into her body. She developed a special "holding tank" inside her where she could detox what she was picking up, sort through it, and decide what was useful and what was not. It taught her a lot about how to process unfamiliar experiences in small doses.

Mingmen Passage

Your Mingmen Passage is the counterpart to your Umbilical Passage. Just as your umbilicus was a link to your mother's nourishment, the Mingmen Passage is the link back to source, back to where you came from as a spirit choosing to have an embodied experience. It is, in short, a passage *home*.

Your Mingmen Passage, when it is intact, anchors at the surface of your body in the Mingmen area of the spine, on your back behind the belly button, between L2–L4 vertebrae. It travels inward from there, making a connection home to the world you are born from: your source.

The Mingmen Passage is a sacred space that is helpful to visit and, if needed, to reinstate. Anyone, who like Dorothy, feels a disconnect from source or who feels lost, like they are an alien in a strange land, or just doesn't feel much at all, most likely has a detached or decimated Mingmen Passage. It is important to keep your passage home open and available to the embodied soul that you are. Otherwise, you might find your Gatekeeper chronically in a defensive or triggered state. For people who experience chronic anxiety or panic, like Dorothy's mother, it is often due to their Gatekeeper reacting to the sense that they won't be able to find their way home.

Clearing the Mingmen Passage improves your access to your inner wisdom and Wiser Self and gives your Storymaker ongoing support in crafting stories that support your soul's purpose.

Guided Visit: Travel Through the Mingmen Passage

With all guided visits, it is important to make sure you are in a safe and comfortable place, with time to explore and let the experience unfold for you. Do whatever preliminary breathing and centering activity you need in order to be present for yourself. See page 13 for instructions on how to access the MP3s.

This visit involves holding and interacting with the Mingmen area on your back at the spine, opposite your belly button. If you can't reach it, you can ask a friend to hold it for you to anchor your journey. Or you can use a favorite piece of clothing or stuffed animal placed under that area as you lie on your back to help you activate and open it.

Before you sit or lie down, flip your hand back and forth a few times, front, then back, on the Mingmen area to unlock any electromagnetic seals your Gatekeeper might have installed to keep people out. (Or ask your friend to do this for you.)

Like all sacred journeys, visits to the Mingmen Passage need to be carried out in safe circumstances, in a secure place where you can do this exploration without distractions. Set an intention to remain for a particular period of time, no longer than half an hour. The purpose of this visit is to open the Mingmen Passage and bring the energies of your "spirit home" into your present life. Get comfortable sitting or lying down, whichever most supports your ability to travel inward.

Gather yourself in by Coming Home: Place one hand on your solar plexus and the other on your heart . . . cross your ankles . . . and breathe in through your nose for three counts, out through your mouth for five counts, taking at least three deep breaths. . . .

Release that hold and reach around your back to hold your Mingmen area with your open hand or fingertips. Breathe in through your nose . . . and out through your mouth, for a series of at least three deep breaths, while holding this spot.

Now, you can release the hold if it is uncomfortable, or continue to hold it. Sink your attention down through the Mingmen opening into the passage behind it (inside you). Just sense what you find there. . . . You may find yourself in a kind of tube or tunnel attached at that spot, or you may find yourself in some other kind of space. Just notice what you pick up about this place. Continue to breathe in through your nose and out through your mouth.

For many people, this passageway is detached or altogether missing. Do what you can to reattach it. Or call on the Universal Support Team to bring you a new one and anchor it at your Mingmen area. Keep your attention focused there, where the Mingmen Passage attaches, until you feel you have secured it to the Mingmen area of your spine.

Now, you are going to investigate this new or reinstated passage using all your senses. Don't worry if you don't see clearly or you can't pick up a lot of detail. Just work with what comes to you and ask for guides or helpers to assist in your efforts.

What kind of shape is your Mingmen Passage in? If it is disturbed, torn, clogged, or otherwise disrupted, take some time, with the help of the Universal Support Team, to reinstate it so it can serve as a healthy inner passage for you. For some people, this can happen as quickly as the thought. For others, you may find yourself using your other hand to physically signal the repair and patching that you need.

At any time, when you feel that is enough for one visit, you can concentrate on your breath, return to the feel of your hand on the Mingmen area, and leave the rest for another day.

If you are ready to travel your passage, follow along it to the other end, wherever that leads you. There is no one right way to do this. Just use your instincts to follow the passage and see where it goes. Although you are roughly inside your body, you may also feel yourself to be in another kind of space altogether. However it works for you, follow this passage to the other end, asking it to guide you to the entrance to your passage home.

The entrance might be a bridge, a tunnel, a doorway, or something else. Look for where it is supposed to lead (it does not always correspond to a physical location in your body) and ask the Universal Support Team to help you get this end of your Mingmen attached firmly to your passage home.

Once you are satisfied that your Mingmen Passage is fully reinstated, you can stop your journey there and return back to the Mingmen area of your spine, or you can continue to explore, crossing the bridge or entering your passage home.

If you choose to continue with a visit *home*, set a little symbolic marker there that reminds you of one thing you want to stay in this life for: a loved one, a pet, to see a place you yearn to visit, or anything else that has meaning for you. Doing this will facilitate your journey back into your body consciousness.

Now, if you have chosen to cross the bridge, pass through the tunnel, or go through the doorway you have found, ask your Councils to meet you on the other side. This is a sacred visit home, and it is not meant to be a leap into other worlds. Instead, stay in the area just on the other side of your bridge, tunnel, or doorway.

This is a wonderful place to get guidance or enlist helpers. If there is an issue you are wishing to resolve, a situation you want to understand, or an aspect of your life you need help with, call upon your Councils and upon the World Wise Web to send you what you need. This is not like asking a genie for three wishes. You are not asking for riches or possessions here. (For example, if you believe money will make you secure, ask for security!) Instead, you are assembling the supports you need, from this source, to nourish and fuel you.

When you are ready to return to body consciousness (or even if you don't want to leave but have been in this place for a while), thank the guides and helpers you have met there and return back across the bridge or through the tunnel or doorway. Travel back along the Mingmen Passage to your energetic spine. If you wish, place your hand again on your Mingmen area. Take at least three deep breaths in through your nose and out through your mouth to bring your attention fully back into your body, your earth elemental self, your physical home.

* * *

When Dorothy first explored her Mingmen Passage, she discovered it was disconnected and utterly trashed. She asked her body if it could be repaired or needed to be replaced. She got a clear sense that she needed a replacement. So she asked the Universal Support Team to bring her one and got it installed fairly easily. She traveled through it to the other side but did not feel ready to cross the bridge home. Still, when she was fully back in her everyday awareness, she said, "I feel totally different. Calmer. Grounded and solid." Her breathing was easier somehow, and in her subsequent visits, she got to know her source, her home, and cultivated it as a place to visit for renewal. Each visit left her feeling increasingly more alive and sourced.

SAFETY NET

Your Safety Net is made up of everything that has touched your heart, that has contributed to your sense of meaning in life. It looks like a big fisherman's net surrounding your body. If it is intact, it supports you and acts like a backup battery. I suspect it is related to what we call our second wind. It also relates to the system Donna Eden calls the minor grid, which is a weave that supports your baseline grid that is like the foundation on a house.

When you are working long hours, pushing through fatigue and resistance, often you will dip into your Safety Net for extra energy and inspiration. This makes sense. It is like a bank account, where day after day you have deposited your joy, your sense of fulfillment, and your sense of meaning, and it becomes a repository you can call on when the resources of a given moment run out. However, it is possible to overuse your Safety Net, drain it, bruise it, and cause it to detach and become inaccessible, so it is an important energy structure to augment and maintain over time. Think about taking a few minutes out of your busy afternoon for the renewal of watching the sunset, of a refreshing walk, or of a quick love exchange with a friend. Everything that feeds you emotionally, spiritually, artistically, and energetically helps keep your Safety Net healthy and ready to catch you when you fall.

Dorothy happened to come see me shortly after I had returned from a trip to Mexico. I had fallen in love with a rainbow hammock I saw there and bought one to cart home with me in my already overstuffed luggage. It was set up on the porch outside my consulting room. When Dorothy said she was not feeling her successes, I took a look at her Safety Net. It was gray and saggy, with big tears in it, and looked like it couldn't hold much. Out of the corner of my eye, I saw my shiny new rainbow hammock, looking a lot like a healthy Safety Net, so on impulse, I said, "Come try out my rainbow hammock."

We had energy tested several of Dorothy's energy systems already and knew that her energies weren't communicating with one another. She was a good sport and immediately agreed to try out the rainbow hammock. As she lay there, she got a beatific look on her face as if a whole tropical vacation were transferring to her body. And, within moments, her Safety Net began to weave and repair itself, taking on the rainbow colors and strengthening all around her.

Needless to say, she was in no hurry to get out of that hammock. Her energy systems were all testing strong and active. And she felt a kind of deep satiation that food had never really given her. She was on her phone, ordering herself a rainbow hammock, before we even had time to discuss what had happened.

If you don't happen to have a rainbow hammock handy, you can use any cloth that has a weave to it and that is large enough to surround your body when lying down, like a blanket, Afghan, or large tablecloth. Place it on your bed or any surface where you can lie on it. If you happen to have something printed in rainbow colors (e.g., a scarf or piece of clothing), place it on the cloth and lie on top of both. (Since a hammock bends to your body, you can either wrap the cloth around you, use an actual hammock, or place your weave in a rocking chair or recliner to give yourself that sense of being held.)

Tune in to the weave of the cloth, the colors, and let them speak to your Safety Net. Then, if you wish, you can invoke in your mind moments of meaning, things that have touched your heart and soul, that have enriched your life. You can bring them into your weave with you—picture that sunset, that perfect day in spring, that time when you couldn't stop laughing with your friend, and so forth—and feel it entering your weave and "juicing" you up.

As you lie there, feeling supported, assess whether there are places in your Safety Net that feel bruised or weak or torn in some way. Trace a five-pointed star and circle (see page 110) over that area to reinstate the weave of elements, the building blocks of your Safety Net. Immersing your Safety Net into another weave, especially one that is colorful and energized like a rainbow hammock, is an excellent recharge for your backup battery. It is also an excellent activity for people who are recovering from a long illness or who are emerging from a time when they have been drained emotionally or because of overwork. It is an excellent renewal tool for caregivers who are better at giving than taking in.

STEERING: NAVIGATING YOUR STORYLINES

Dorothy had a list of things she always wanted: to lose weight, to be recognized at work, and to get a position where she could lead others and be creative. She used these as goals to navigate toward. But then she achieved them and found herself at a standstill, not sure where to go next. Wisely, she responded to her lack of wind to take some time, to look at what her ship needed, and to repair her equipment.

If you find yourself setting destinations and not getting there or enjoying the travel, you would also probably benefit from some upgrades on your equipment for navigating this life: In general, that means working with your Storymaker and Gatekeeper; in particular, it means making sure your steering mechanisms are in working order.

In the context of creating and living storylines, *steering* has to do with perspective and discernment: How do you see where you are and where you are headed? How do you evaluate your choices? We usually think of these as functions of your brain. But, in fact, there are several physical and energetic tools to help you navigate in life. They affect not only your physical balance and processing, but also how your mind processes inputs from the world *out there*. These include your Assemblage Point, your tailbone, your face and nose, your heart and gut areas, and your third eye and gaze.

Assemblage Point (AP)

The term "Assemblage Point" was borrowed by Donna Eden from shaman Carlos Castaneda to refer to a gathering point in your energies, where the strands of your nature come together and form a glowing ball of light in front of your heart, usually about an arm's length ahead of you. Donna describes this as a North Star, guiding you in life and guiding you home after death. I see it as the lady on the prow of the ship. If she is positioned correctly, you can steer toward her, and she guides you forward. If she is leaning left or right, shattered in pieces, or not visible, your ship easily steers off course. (See Protocol: Course Correction on page 195 for techniques to reassemble your Assemblage Point and adjust your steering mechanism.)

If your AP is out of alignment or shattered, you can experience all kinds of distortion of perception. One client I worked with was gushing about and planning to vote for a candidate who, from my perspective, contradicted many of my client's values. I couldn't understand why she was so gung ho. In the course of our session, we reassembled and repositioned her AP, and as she was preparing to leave, she said, "You know, I have no idea why I thought that candidate was so great. I'm not going to vote for them. I don't know what I was thinking!"

Tailbone

The tailbone, or coccyx, acts as a rudder for your body to orient in space and keep itself upright. But it also ties in to your Assemblage Point, and when it is out of alignment, it can pull your AP, the lady on the prow of your ship, off-balance as well.

Face and Nose

Think about the phrase, "I can't face it." Although your face is designed to swivel and turn, when you are ready to decide or act, facing forward will help you orient the body and your storyline to support where you are headed. Facing forward supports your sense of motivation. Play with this for a moment:

1. Name something you are unclear about, trying to decide, or wanting clarity on, saying: "I want insight into . . . (e.g., *how to get my taxes done more comfortably)*": First say this facing forward, just feeling into the issue.

2. Turn your face downward, toward the floor, say your phrase, and sense into what arises.

3. Turn your head to the left and repeat the phrase. Note how you feel and what you think.

4. Now angle your face upward, facing the ceiling, and repeat the phrase. Tune in to how this affects your inquiry.

5. Repeat the phrase facing right, and notice what arises.

6. Now, facing forward again, repeat the phrase once more, and see how your perspective has changed or shifted, or whether you feel a shift in motivation.

Similarly, try saying the phrase again, first, while cutting off air to your nose and breathing through your mouth. Then, release your hold and breathe in through your nose while asking, "Give me insight into . . ."

Heart and Gut Areas

We have an energetic band around our heart area and navigation receptors in our gut area designed to help us steer and discern truth: It is no accident that when we want to claim inner knowing, we say, "I know it in my heart" or "I know it in my gut."

When you are feeling confused, you can say, "I'd like insight into *[name your confusion]*." Hold first your heart band with a hand on each side of your chest at the level of your heart and activate your heart wisdom. Similarly, hold your gut area with both hands, side by side, and repeat the query, "I'd like insight into . . ." This will activate the steering mechanism and knowing in your gut.

Third Eye and Gaze

Your gaze and third eye (which sits midway between and extends above your eyebrows) form a triangle that helps stabilize your view of things. Like the Assemblage Point, when your gaze is out of alignment (literally and figuratively), too far in the distance or turned inward or back to the past, canting left or right or too far up or down, it will distort your thinking and understanding.

To be clear, your steering equipment is designed to move, to be able to pull in information from all the directions, and support you in creating your chosen routes and storylines in life. So the goal isn't to keep them front and center. But forward motion requires them to move and return to center, to *be centered*, if you want to be living healthy stories and facing your truth.

Take a moment to think about some storyline you are living. Maybe you're feeling a partner isn't *there* for you, maybe you are worried you've taken a wrong turn, or maybe you want to validate a goal you've set before you commit resources to it. Maybe it is someone else's storyline or a cultural belief that you suspect is pulling you off your path or distorting your perceptions.

Write out your thoughts about that topic (or record them or share them with an exploration buddy). Then try the Course Correction protocol to follow, and afterward, retell the storyline or concern, jotting down how you now perceive it or think about it. If there is no change, wait twenty-four hours and check in a third time. Sometimes your body will need a night's sleep to reboot before it can register the changes to the equipment.

Protocol: Course Correction

Note: You don't need to do all the course corrections in this protocol at once. You can work with righting your ship over time.

Adjusting Your AP

Reassemble your AP using a Harmonizing Hook-Up, which is best done in silence for at least three minutes:

1. Place one hand flat on your left pelvic bone (next to your left hip) and your other hand flat on the front of your left shoulder (covering where your arm attaches to your torso).

2. Imagine yourself in a rainbow hammock (or literally wrap yourself in a rainbow weave) and breathe in through your nose and out through your mouth.

A Harmonizing Hook-Up will strengthen your Body Weave, your Safety Net, and finally, when your deep weaves feel more intact, bring your Assemblage Point back together and into position at arm's length out in front of your heart.

If you do not feel certain your AP has completely reassembled and come home or that it will stay put, you can hold the Harmonizing Hook-Up longer than three minutes, even up to half an hour. This is also great to do in bed over several evenings to reinforce the message that it is safe to hold together and steer your own course.

Loosening your gas cap(s) (see page 100) and adjusting your tailbone (see next section) can also help your AP to reassemble and come home to its proper position.

Resetting Your Rudder

Your tailbone acts as a rudder to your ship; it also affects the tension in all the "lines" that form your Assemblage Point. Sometimes adjusting the tailbone will allow you to shift the tensions and conflicts within your story-line or perceptions.

1. Adjust or micro-adjust your tailbone to make sure it is able to move freely *and* in position to steer properly. To adjust your tailbone (while standing): Rub your hands together to activate the energy centers in them. Then place either hand over your tailbone, letting the warmth seep into the area. Invite all the muscles that hold your sacrum and tailbone in place to just relax and melt into that warmth.

2. Use your palm chakra, the energy vortex in your palm, as a kind of magnet to create a link with your tailbone: Inhale, and on the exhale, gently guide your tailbone into correct position, using your intuition and the knowing in your hand to determine where it is and where it needs to be. You may need to do a series of gentle micro-adjustments rather than a single pull.

Resetting Your Face and Nose

1. Place both hands on your face, cradling it (holding your Storymaker anchors), and align your little fingers so they each point to a center of the eye they are near. Your little fingers help ground you via your embodiment stream (stomach meridian).

2. Throughout steps 3 to 8, continue to cradle your face, while you breathe in through your nose and out through your mouth, and make small movements to loosen your neck muscles, keeping your torso facing forward.

3. Roll your head gently forward, so your face is parallel to the floor. Breathe deeply. Do your best to keep your neck loose.

4. Now, bring your head back to center, facing forward, and take a big breath in through your nose and out through your mouth. Again, move your head gently to help release your neck muscles.

5. Still cradling, turn your face to the left and breathe deeply. Loosen your neck muscles. Then bring your face back to center.

6. Turn your cradled face to the right, and again, breathe deeply and adjust your neck muscles. Then return to center, taking a deep breath.

7. Turn your cradled face upward, toward the heavens. Breathe in what this direction brings to you. Loosen your neck muscles, exhale fully, and then bring your cradled face back to center.

8. Remove your hands from your face and take several deep breaths facing forward, allowing your head to bob gently, finding its balance, and settling its weight to rest easily and centered on the column of your neck.

Activating Your Heart and Gut Knowing

1. Interlace your fingers, and place your joined hands over your heart area, across both the left and right sides of your chest. Breathe in through your nose, out through your mouth, and feel your hands and heart establish contact and converse. Keep this hold until you feel your knowing is centered in your heart.

2. Then, repeat this over your gut area. With interlaced fingers, cover as much of your lower gut area as you can. Breathe deeply and slowly, allowing your hands and gut to establish contact and converse. Keep this hold until you feel your knowing is centered in your gut.

3. Finally, end by holding your heart and gut together in a hook-up hold to align their knowing into unity.

Activating Your Third Eye and Gaze

1. Shut your eyes, and trace a five-pointed star and circle (see page 110) over your third eye, on your forehead. Start on the bottom left side of the star (the star in this case is "printed" on your forehead, so the element water is over your right eyebrow).

   Trace on your skin between water and fire, fire and metal, metal and wood, wood and earth, and earth and water, and then circle around (starting above your right eyebrow, upward, left, down, and back to your starting point). This helps elementally balance your vision and your perspective.

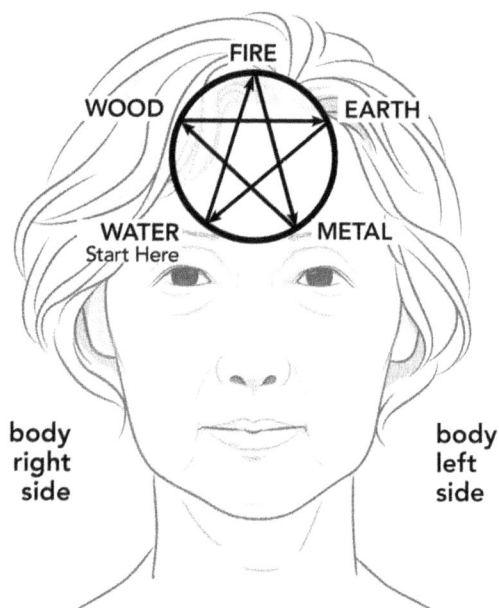

Figure 7.1.

2. Still with eyes shut, go to the center of each line of the star you just traced, and stretch *from the center toward each of the points*:

   - Stretch the water-fire connection.

   - Stretch the fire-metal connection.

   - Stretch the metal-wood connection.

   - Stretch the wood-earth connection.

   - Stretch the earth-water connection.

   Then tap along the circle to activate more energy flow.

3. Open your eyes, and gaze ahead of you. Soften your gaze, no strain, just letting in whatever enters your eyes. Breathe deeply. Then in turn, gaze softly left, up, right, and down.

4. Shut your eyes and look back at your past at a moment when you felt present and alive. (If you can't think of one, imagine yourself in a setting where you could feel present and alive.) Then gently, with eyes still shut, look forward into your future, your field of possibility, to gaze at something that catches your eye. Don't strain. Just invite something in your potential to come to your attention. If you can't think of anything, focus on your next breath, and *watch* it, with eyes shut, enter your nose and travel into your lungs.

5. Open your eyes, and if you want, you can now revisit any situation you were feeling unbalanced by before to see how your perspective has shifted.

• • •

When you learn to dive beneath the story to work with your Storymaker, you will discover that you can heal the parts of your story that weren't responding to self-talk or efforts to program new behaviors or resolutions of change.

Learning to partner with your Storymaker; to *anchor, frame,* and set the terms of engagement; *weave* your web of meaning; *source* the nourishment you need; and improve your ability to set and *steer* a course is deep healing work. But it does not need to be complex or heavy. Any step in any of the protocols in this (and my other books) can stand alone as an in-the-moment dialogue with the mechanism your consciousness uses to creates your life: your Storymaker. Storymaker *loves* conversation and responds as most of us creatures do to overtures of friendship and affection.

But what about all those old stories, painful experiences, traumas, and feelings still clogging your mind and heart, still causing your ship's autopilot to run away with you? As I mentioned earlier, your Storymaker is designed to *learn*—the sixth task of your Storymaker—to distill meaning from experience and create energy templates that run your autopilot and codify your own personal take on reality.

In the next two chapters, we'll explore how you can *unlearn* those templates and how to clear and rewrite your story at various dimensions of your being. Being able to heal and co-create your stories will alter your life and provide the awakening most appropriate to your soul's truth.

CHAPTER EIGHT

Track and Heal Your Stories

Aviva spent the past year dealing with the boss from hell and was thinking seriously of leaving her job. She referred to her boss as the "bitch witch" and felt belittled and constantly criticized by this woman, even after Aviva had done something perfectly competent. "I have had this job for eleven years, and for the first ten of them, I thought of it as my dream job. Then I got this new boss, and I don't see how I can stay. I'm looking for insight into what's going on with this situation!"

We were in a workshop where energy medicine students were learning how to track and balance stories through the dimensions of their being. I had asked the students to just go around the circle and share what they wanted to track. I presented it like this: "Put your inquiry into the pot, so we can get ideas about what everyone here is exploring." In other words, this was not a discussion. But, immediately, another student jumped in and said, "Maybe she's racist."

Aviva was more courteous than I might have been. "I suppose that's possible," she said, "but I doubt it. She's Arab American too." Her fellow student looked ready to debate, so I jumped in and reminded them, "Let's just hear each person's topic without comment. The whole point of tracking our stories in this protocol is to learn from the *energies* about what is going on and how we might address it."

The fellow student meant well—she wanted to support Aviva politically against what the student immediately wrote into the story: racism. And it might have been true. But it is also true that we often jump in to interpret or rewrite other people's stories from our own perspectives, rather than listening and asking questions about what *they* have experienced. And, perhaps worse, our minds are schooled in today's culture to jump into our *own* stories with psychological or sociological or groupthink political explanations that, while sometimes true, can flatten our experiences into stereotypes or totally miss the boat. Lived experience is richer and fuller than most of our minds can encompass, in part because we don't give ourselves time and space to explore and investigate and fully *live* our experiences and let them teach us on their own terms.

In the hands-on practice time, Aviva and her practice partner used the phrase "this situation with my boss" to help Aviva track where this storyline lived within her and what all it entailed in energetic terms. Working together, they brought in Radiance to clear the templates of experience that Aviva's Storymaker had set up in response to her encounters with the bitch witch. They collected insights and balanced her story using energy medicine, as they'd just learned in class, at each level of Aviva's being.

After the practice time, the students took a fifteen-minute break, and Aviva returned to the group discussion with a peculiar look on her face. I invited students to share their experiences with the protocol, and when Aviva got a chance to speak, she pulled out her cell phone, saying, "About twenty minutes after my partner and I finished tracking and balancing my story, I got this email." It was from her boss, and it started with: "I owe you a huge apology. I have been really unkind and unfair to you this year." The boss went on to explain briefly what had been going on for her and promised to be vigilant, to stop taking it out on Aviva. She gave Aviva permission to speak up if she noticed the unfair behaviors creeping back in.

Stunned silence! For most of the students in the workshop, this was a *Twilight Zone* moment. How could Aviva influence her boss by tracking her own story? One student asked me, "Do you think this is just a coincidence?"

"No," I told her, "unless by *co-incidence* you mean two interrelated incidents. We are wired together in our stories with other characters, and when we change how our energies participate, it can shift the story for everyone."

I had been using this protocol with clients and teaching it in workshops for some time by then, and, in fact, it was quite common to see quick shifts in a dynamic, to hear from other people involved and see a change in their attitudes or choices, to notice sticky behaviors drop away, and even to have physical symptoms clear up with almost unbelievable speed.

KEYS TO THE KINGDOM

When I first discovered this way of working, I felt like I'd been given the keys to the kingdom. And perhaps I had. This isn't just a magic recipe: *Do these seven steps and then you'll heal.* It's a way of working with your energies that involves tracking the energy storyline and interacting with it *where it lives.*

Up until then, when I'd ask for insight, I'd sit at the surface of my awareness, in my body, or up in my head. And I'd expect insight to rise into my brain like the messages in one of those Magic 8 Balls we used to play with as kids. Are you familiar with those? You ask a question, shake the Magic 8 Ball, and one of twenty preprogrammed answers floats into the viewing screen— Outlook good: *It is certain; You may rely on it; Signs point to yes,* or Outlook bad: *Don't count on it; My sources say no,* or Outlook neutral: *Reply hazy, Try again; Better not tell you now.*

But when my Councils taught me to travel in the Country of the Mind and through the dimensions of self, I learned that I could track a storyline to where it lived and discover all of what my being had learned and codified about the topic. I could bring healing to the places where the problems and imbalances were causing me grief. I could co-write the stories where they lived and see very different expressions in my body, mind, emotions, and lived experiences as a result.

And that's the essence of Storyline Track and Balance. Is not just a fix, though often you will get amazing results. It is also a form of inquiry, exploration, dialogue, and awakening. And it can frame any other energy medicine (or self-therapy) you want to do. It involves using some of the tools and practices you've already learned in this book:

1. Traveling within the dimensions of your being to track your story (in this chapter, we will focus on traveling within the levels of the chakras).

2. Assessing what you find there, expressing itself in the language of energy.

3. Dialoguing with what you find there, using the language of energy.

4. Bringing Radiance via the Divine Hook-Up (see page 37) to clear or balance templates (which are energy storage for your learning and experience).

5. Asking for helpers, such as the Universal Support Team, your Councils, and/or guides from the World Wise Web to step in and supply resources and help with repairs.

6. Doing simple energy medicine to shift the energy dynamics.

7. Planting seeds of change in places deep within you where the soil is fertile for change.

WHAT IS AN ENERGY TEMPLATE?

If it is true, as scientists have claimed, that you replace the cells of your body, on average, every seven years, why do you still have a scar or chronic illness in year eight? What tells the clusters of cells that make up your body to hold on to whatever storyline of damage, malfunction, or imbalance is expressed through your physical body? For that matter, what is it in each of us telling our cells how to behave, telling our organs to regenerate or not, telling our skin to knit evenly or with jagged scar tissue, and so forth?

I know pop-science thinking says blithely, "DNA." And more thoughtful science writers are tracing the chemical mechanisms of learning coded into the cells. But my Councils suggested another mechanism that I find extremely useful because it is something I—and you—can readily work with that will influence what happens with our body and mind.

It is a mechanism within your subtle energies, a function of your Storymaker, that codifies each experience into energy structures I call templates.

A template is a little energy map, a guidepost to how energies should behave in certain circumstances. From the moment you begin to form a body-mind self in this life, each time you have an experience, your Storymaker forms an energy template to encode what you are learning—positive and negative and everything in between. Some of that learning is wired into the brain and its functions, for sure, because your brain is a major center for processing experience and for thinking. But all your learning, experience, and storylines also get encoded into energy templates and stored throughout your being to guide the behaviors of the energies you are made of.

I am not the most visual of visionaries, but to me, energy templates look a bit like little five-element glyphs, with a star and circle, but with the arms of the star in all kinds of crazy positions, and the spaces of the glyph rich with something that feels suspiciously like "meaning" when I tune in to them. I asked another, more visual energy friend what templates looked like to her after I described what they looked like to me, and she said, "Absolutely, they look like that to me too." So, there's a sample of two. I'm not sure it matters what they look like because you can learn to work with them, even if you don't ever see energy and only perceive it through some kind of abstract knowing in your head.

But you may find it useful to have a visual image of the little five-element discs distributed throughout your energy systems because it is part of this protocol to use the five-element glyph to help open up conversation with your stored experiences (see Figure 8.1).

The name "templates" fits because they are not just recordings of past experience. They aren't memories. They are distilled understand-

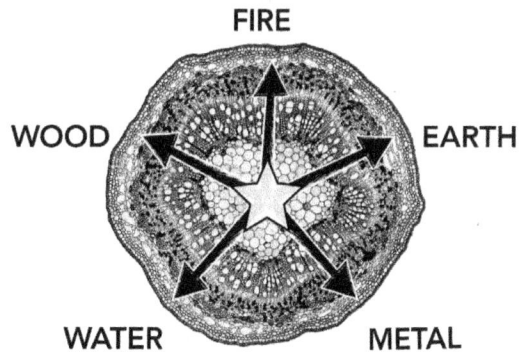

Figure 8.1. Five-Element Discs

ings meant to guide your behaviors and choices going forward from the time they were formed. Templates offer guidance to your Gatekeeper and auto-pilot on what to fund (energetically), what to avoid, where to put resources (physical and mental), and how and why. And often what's coded into them is the storyline: your understandings and thoughts and feelings about this experience that will influence you going forward.

Templates can both serve and hamper you. For example, you're two years old, in your yard, and a neighbor's dog runs up to you, perhaps trying to get you to play. She leaps up and accidentally pushes you over, being nearly as big as you are. You are frozen with terror, and your mom, who is talking to the neighbor, says over her shoulder, "You're okay." The neighbor calls the dog off. And your Storymaker forms a template, storing it in your root chakra, with copies in your solar plexus chakra and throat chakra. Encoded into it is an instruction to "freeze" when something big and scary comes at you. It encodes also a slight aversion to dogs (is that why you became a cat person?) and an instruction to feel unsafe and suspicious when someone tells you that you're okay when you don't feel okay. Also encoded into that template are instructions to the Gatekeeper and autopilot about how to move chemicals and hormones in the face of similar encounters.

Someone else's Storymaker might make a very different template or might respond differently to the dog in that moment, depending on experiences from this and other lifetimes and what purpose the event serves in that soul's evolution (also depending on how their parent, neighbor, and the world around them react). So they might have templates that tell their Gatekeeper to respond with a massive allergic response (aversion) or its opposite (attraction), a yearning to get to know all dogs as possible playmates.

We don't just record our traumas; we record all kinds of experience, and it makes our life richer and more meaningful because we have ongoing storylines that build on our past experiences. From an energetic perspective, trauma is, for the most part, energy templates that don't serve us, keeping our Gatekeepers reacting to painful storylines that keep getting renewed in *year eight*. Painful experiences for which we have cleared the templates are just that: painful memories. Not trauma.

Perhaps templates relate to body memory in the sense that they store data to guide the body and mind. But they are also like brain memory in that experiences register and are stored in very individual ways and influence our storymaking and gatekeeping as we move forward. And they are a bit like the concept of "subconscious" because they can encode both very complex and very basic information that we don't always realize we are encoding.

Although early templates can be potent and sometimes make it seem like our inner infant and child are driving the ship, we continue to make new templates throughout our lives and update existing ones.

Fran, who also attended one of my Storyline Track and Balance workshops, wanted to track templates for being hard of hearing. She was curious if it could help, because she struggled in group situations to follow what people were saying. She and her practice partner tracked the templates through her solar plexus chakra. That was what showed up as the ripest place to explore the storyline. (I'll show you how to do this later in this chapter.) I noticed at one point that Fran was sitting bolt upright, looking stunned.

Her practice partner waved at me frantically, and when I got to them, her partner said, "We just cleared templates for Fran's hearing issue, and she says now she can hear what those two"—she pointed to the people about twenty feet away—"are saying."

Fran said, "It's like the volume button just got turned up. I think I'm hearing normally now."

I encouraged them to test it with an experiment. The practice partner tried whispering while turning her head so Fran couldn't read her lips, and Fran could hear her. She tried saying things at various volumes and pitches. Needless, to say, their classmates got interested and helped suggest some testing. Everyone was happy for Fran, congratulating her. I noticed that Fran looked a bit like a deer in the headlights.

The next day in class, we did some sharing about what changes people had noticed as a result of clearing their templates. Fran seemed subdued, and when it came time for her to speak, she said, "All last evening, my hearing worked great. I went out to dinner with some friends and could actually hear what they were saying, despite the noise in the restaurant—for the first time in years! But then before bed, I called my husband to tell him about it. He's hearing impaired too, and I thought he'd be excited about it. But he said, 'Are you still going to love me if you can hear and I can't?' I assured him I would and that we could try to clear his templates too. But when I woke up this morning, my hearing was back to what it was. It didn't hold. I don't think I was ready to hear if my husband couldn't."

In fact, the template clearing probably did hold. Once you clear a template, it is cleared. But Fran's Storymaker, in response to her husband's reaction, had set up a new template to replace the one she had cleared. This one tied her deafness into her husband's more explicitly. Our energies are bound to those we love, not just because we are codependent emotionally but because we are wired together energetically and via our Storymakers. Her Storymaker had gone ahead and created a new template to reflect her ambivalence about leaving her hard-of-hearing buddy behind by being able to hear again.

The class suggested ways to work around this: mostly by clearing his templates. But Fran said, "For now, I'm going to see how this unfolds. I think I've got other templates in me that I will need to explore before I can be certain I won't just make a new one to block my hearing."

Not only do we make new templates as we move through life but also sometimes the old ones still serve a significant purpose. So tracking is not just a matter of clearing them; it is also about letting them teach us what that purpose is so we can address it in other ways.

You might be asking at this point, "If we make so many templates, doesn't it get crowded in there?" Yes, it does, and often we have contradictory templates: the one that says avoid dogs, and the one that says, "My partner loves dogs, so I need to stay open." This can be very confusing to the body and create stress that is hard to release. In the normal course of things, some templates get stored and don't activate very often; others are more likely to come up and try to steer the ship. Templates can fade and become inert on their own. Sometimes a new experience will get codified in such a way that the old one just dies off. For example, if your first experience of riding a bike was mixed (it was both fun and scary), you might have a template encoding that ambivalence. But if you subsequently have a lot of fun riding your bike, maybe with friends who love it, your Storymaker is likely to overwrite or erase the original template. End of story.

But if you feel your reality is clogged, torqued, or limited by past experience, tracking and balancing your storyline is an important skill set. Templates can easily be cleared or balanced out, and that is often necessary self-care.

Clearing templates does not erase them from your memory! For example, you might remember you didn't love bike riding at first. But it is not at this point a guidepost template and has probably just been subsumed into your new bike-loving template as a little energetic nuance.

Templates are rich and fascinating (to me at least), and I could probably write a whole book about them. But, for now, here are some observations about them in more abbreviated form:

1. Templates don't each operate independently. Your Storymaker groups them into storylines . . . and often the theme is energetic rather than logical: Instead of "all my templates about dogs," the group might be, "all those times I felt scared by something new and unexpected." That's why you can react to co-workers as if they were family members and associate strangers with your ex!

2. There is some logic to where various templates get stored. The chakras are one of the richest energy-storage systems, but you can also have templates stored in your body at the location of an injury or insult. For example, we often have templates stored in our face relating to how others have reacted to us. We also store templates in a master blueprint I call the *harmonic self*. (We'll visit that in chapter 9.) But since templates are grouped and linked, you can often find a single place within the chakras to clear all of them in the grouping. You don't need to chase down each individual template.

3. Templates are complex and nuanced. Sometimes you will want to track and balance them *not* to clear them but merely to balance them, update them, and clear out instructions that don't fit your current conscious choices.

4. Your soul distills experience and is nourished by it, but as far as I can tell, you don't take templates with you when you die. They dissolve when your consciousness no longer animates your body. Therefore, you aren't carrying your traumas and gripes with you, even though the soul may choose lifetimes that help it balance out painful experiences in this life with experiences in another life that bring more diverse perspectives.

5. Templates form the basis of habits. The first time you do something, it is an experience. The second time you do it, your former experience influences your choices. The more you do it, the more the template holds the "habit." For good habits, like brushing your teeth or hair, having a

positive template tilting you toward continuing the experience is useful. You are supported (groomed) to keep the behavior. If it's a negative template, it can make self-care difficult or impossible. I knew a young woman with aversion to brushing her teeth, stemming from a time when her teeth were sensitive, and she was unable to find a workaround. In that young woman's case, her teeth all rotted and needed to be pulled. It was tragic that she didn't know how to clear her unproductive templates.

When you track templates, are you encountering your truth? Yes and no. You are tracking your *experience, thoughts, past conclusions,* and *internalized beliefs.* When you say, "Experience has taught me" or "I've learned from experience," you are really saying, "Here's how my Storymaker codified that experience."

Is the template true? Not necessarily. It may still be true for you but not fit for others. Or it might not even fit for you now. Much of it was your historical interpretation, often created by your much younger self when you were knocked off-balance, when you were yearning for certain outcomes, or in response to other people's Storymakers influencing your interpretations. It is quite possibly not the truth you would choose today, even if it feels like reality.

In this time when we are challenged to discern truth, we need to be able to recognize that our cherished truth (and other people's cherished truths) might rest on distorted storylines, socialization we've had in things that aren't necessarily true, and a sheer accumulation of conflicting templates that keep us from accessing our own consciousness for guidance. Sometimes, it gets so crowded in there. With so many guideposts, we can't easily hear or recognize inner guidance or reliable outer validation.

TRACKING AND BALANCING YOUR TEMPLATES

The process of tracking and balancing your templates includes getting insight into what you have concluded based on your experience. It also includes learning what filters you put on your experience going forward, based on those conclusions. This experiential knowing may need to be updated with the light of consciousness, with Radiance. And that's at the root of the Storyline Track and Balance process.

We'll look at each step in the process, but please remember, this is a travel guide, not a recipe. You can adjust your own Storyline Track and Balance work to your particular situation. Depending on how much time you have, you might make a quick info-finding, light-bringing visit, or indulge in a longer, more thorough, more nuanced healing session. This is also a great process to do with a friend.

There's more detail to follow to help you understand the prompts, but here are the steps in overview:*

1. Do some simple energy medicine to calm your Gatekeeper and center your Storymaker.

2. Frame your inquiry (come up with a name for what you are tracking).

3. Select the chakra where you will track the issue.

4. State your goal: "Show me all templates related to *[your inquiry name]*," and travel down to the first level of your chosen chakra.

5. Trace each arm of the five-pointed star on your chosen chakra to tune in to (and activate) the elemental balance.

6. Track and balance the energies.

7. Do the Divine Hook-Up on page 37 to bring Radiance into the conversation.

8. Explore what you find in this space.

9. Call upon helpers, guides, the Universal Support Team, or your Councils to help you repair the space or rewrite the storyline.

---

* These instructions are for doing this protocol for yourself or supporting a friend to do it. For professional healers, who use energy testing and have some grounding in Eden Energy Medicine, I have a full video course, downloadable from https://listening-in.com/digitalstore/ or available on DVD.

10. Do energy medicine as needed to balance your energies here where they live, relative to your inquiry.

11. When you feel the energies are balanced at this level, trace the five-pointed star and circle (see page 110) to help *seal the deal.*

12. Put out your palm and ask your guides for seeds to plant in the space that support your highest good.

13. Return to the surface to jot down or record what you experienced.

14. Then proceed to the next level down in the same chakra, and repeat steps 4–9, using the same inquiry.

15. Once you have tracked your issue through all levels of the self (all the levels of the chakra) you can review your notes to interpret what you've discovered.

On page 224, I offer you a Storyline Track and Balance guided visit to walk you through these steps.

First, though, here's a discussion of each of these steps to familiarize you with the process.

1. Do some simple energy medicine to calm your Gatekeeper and center your Storymaker.

While tracking and balancing your energies includes energy medicine at all levels, it helps to get your everyday self calmed and balanced a bit before you begin your journey.

Most of the energy medicine in this book will serve this purpose. I suggest starting with Coming Home (see page 46). Place one hand on your solar plexus, one on your heart, cross your ankles, and do 3-5 breathing. If you are riled up or in reactivity, try doing the Third Eye–Belly Button Hook-Up (see page 38), Porcupine Reset (see page 73), and then Expanding Hearts (see page 72).

2. Frame your inquiry (come up with a name for what you are tracking).

This is important to know: *Tracking your storyline does not require you to relive it.* Tracking a trauma to balance it does not ask you to re-experience or dissect the trauma. You can work on the purely energetic level, drop a little deeper into the metaphoric and symbolic level, or drop into an exploration of whatever storyline presents itself, without needing to enter into the emotions or relive the trauma.

Also, you don't need to already know what's wrong to investigate what's going on. You can say, "Show me templates related to this habit I have of being chronically late," or "Show me templates related to this weird rash," or "Show me templates related to this feeling I can't put my finger on." As long as *you* know more or less what you are talking about, your Storymaker will be able to dialogue with you about it. I've had clients who wanted help tracking an issue but didn't want me to know what it was. I've just asked them to give it a random name, such as "Henry," so we could ask for insight into Henry at each level of the chakra.

When I work with a client, I often ask them to talk for a few minutes about the situation they want to track. Just bringing up parts of it to make sure their Storymaker knows which templates and storyline they want to track. When I do this process with myself, I use shorthand and just know what I'm referring to: "This situation with John," or "These bumps on my back," or "My reactions to the news yesterday."

What can you track for?

◆ Insight into something specific

◆ More general insight when you don't know what's going on

◆ Guidance on how and where to heal something

◆ A chance to bring Radiance into the conversation

◆ A chance to encounter your energies and balance them where they live

◆ To prepare the ground and plant seeds of change where they can make a difference

You can use this process to address *health situations* both specific and vague (e.g., "This rash on my chest" or "My low energy this year").

You can track a *social or relationship issue or habit* (e.g., "Templates relating to my feeling pressure when another person shows interest" or "My constant conflict with Jan about money").

You can investigate *chronic reactivity* (e.g., "I can't stand the smell of fish" or "Templates related to my allergy to dust mites" or "My anger when I feel ignored").

You can look at *addictions/patterns you can't seem to change* (e.g., "Templates relating to compulsive eating" or "My reaction to sibling rivalry").

You can use it to get more insights into your *emotional state* (e.g., "My constant state of being on alert" or "This weird mood I don't understand").

You can look for templates from *early programming* (e.g., "Templates from growing up Baptist" or "Templates related to 'I should always clean my plate'").

It is also helpful to track and balance templates related to *injuries or illness that won't heal* (e.g., "Templates for why my knee won't heal" or "Templates related to these chronic virus symptoms").

One thing you *can't* do is track your templates in generic ways. Jim was on a crash course of self-perfection. He had been an engineer for most of his career and, in his late fifties, had a surprising spiritual awakening. He was training in a number of modalities at once to make up for lost time: energy medicine, shamanism, quantum healing, and others. He tried to track "All my templates for faults in my character." His Storymaker wouldn't cooperate! I suggested he start with tracking "My need to do things perfectly."

3. Select the chakra where you will track the issue.

Although you can track and balance your storyline templates elsewhere, the chakras are particularly rich places to travel. They anchor at our deepest cosmic levels, travel up through the layers of the self, and emanate outward into what I call the "field of possibility." They are energy-transport mechanisms, bathing the organs they travel through. They energize the work of the body and the stories of your Storymaker, and they help create the magnetic aura field around you that filters and calls in experience.

The chakra energies communicate meaning between your deepest self and the world. And because they are swirling energies, like tornados, they can call in or repel experiences. This calling in and repulsion is guided by your Storymaker via the templates.

This may seem very abstract. But, in my mind, it's a bit like a player piano. It is a real piano, but when you put in the piano roll, coded with instructions, it plays a particular song. The templates help guide your energies to play particular songs.

Often your storyline "lives" in several of the chakras. I've even tracked issues that lived in *all* my chakras. But if you find the one that is juiciest, the highest priority to start with, you can usually track and balance there and it will end up clearing and balancing the storyline in the other chakras as well. It is rare that I have to track and balance the same storyline in two separate chakras.

There are a number of ways to determine which chakra is juiciest to travel through to encounter a particular storyline.

♦ You can just place your hand over each chakra in turn and state (out loud if possible): "This is the priority place to track *[name your issue]*." You might hear a yes or no in your head, or you might feel a magnetic pull on your hand that is stronger than at the other chakras. The priority chakra will often exert a discernible pull on your hand (or sinking down of your hand) in response to that statement. Note: It is a statement, not a question. So you are saying, "This is the priority place to track *[my issue with my uncle]*."

♦ You can say, "Show me which chakra is the priority place to track *[name your issue]*," and shut your eyes to see which chakra lights up in your mind's eye.

♦ You can use your intuition, based on the theme of each chakra (see Figure 8.2):

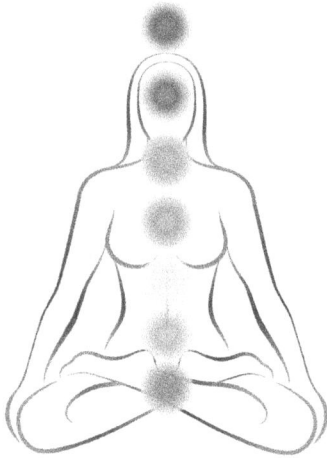

7. Crown: connection to the cosmic mind

6. Third Eye: ability to see inner and outer experiences

5. Throat: communications, expression

4. Heart: heart connections and the ability to take in the Web of Connections

3. Solar plexus: creation of identity and embodiment

2. Sacral: authenticity

1. Root: earthly connections

Figure 8.2. Energetic Priorities of the Seven Chakras

ENERGY TESTING IS NOT NECESSARY

Energy testing is an art form in itself, so if you find it hard to use, don't bother. The energy medicine in this book does not rely on energy testing, and in general, I encourage students to use intuition as their first choice to dialogue with the body.

So, while energy testing is not necessary to locate the priority chakra, if you are already comfortable with energy testing or using a pendulum, this is a situation where limited vocabulary (strong test/weak test or yes/no) can be helpful. See Appendix A for three simple energy self-tests. Personally, I like the Finger Extension Test because I have used it enough to feel confident that I'm getting reliable soundings of the energy.

To energy test for a priority chakra, say, "Show me a weak test if this is the priority place to track *[name your issue]*." Tap twice and energy test. A weak test shows that is the priority place to track; the other chakras should all test strong in response to the same question.

4. Travel down to the first level of your chosen chakra to see if templates for the issue live there.

In chapter 5, I offer you a practice visit to take soundings in the levels of the chakra using an elevator to travel between the floors (see page 136). For many people, this makes travel easy and straightforward. Some of my clients don't like the underground garage image—it feels claustrophobic or just weird to them. So if that's true for you, I encourage you to find whatever passage makes sense at each level.* Just ask to see a passage to carry you from one level to the next, or feel your attention sinking until you find yourself in the next layer down.

The important issue here is that you are traveling from the surface of your body inward to track your storyline. Traveling outward from the body takes you into a different realm that we will explore in chapter 9.

5. Trace each arm of the five-pointed star to tune in to the elemental balance.

Your mind and attention are now at the first level down. Keeping the issue in mind or renaming it out loud (e.g., "This issue *[name your issue]* with my mother"), you are going to trace each arm of the five-pointed star from the center outward, starting with water. For example, if you are tracking in your third chakra, you will be tracing this on your skin at your solar plexus. (See Figure 8.3 on the following page.)

This step is important: It calls up all the elements of the energy story to open the conversation. You can simply do the tracing or use this to get information about which elements need support in the storyline here.

To get information, as you trace each arm of the star, take soundings (or energy test) each element to see whether they need support. A weak test means it needs support! This is useful if you use the five elements as a vocabulary to understand what your energies are doing. If all five elements are out of

---

* This elevator-free configuration was offered by one of my teaching assistants,
Stacy Newman, who has taken Storyline Track and Balance and made it her own.
I encourage you to find the mode of travel most natural and comfortable for you.

balance, I call that "blotto." It means you have fallen apart, relative to this issue, at this level of the chakra. You will need some *honey* or coherence, at the very least.

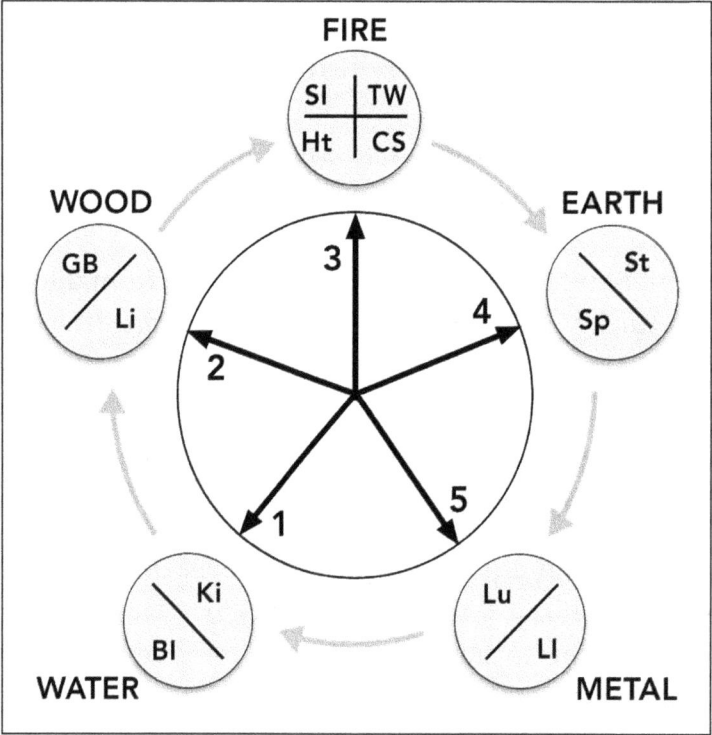

Figure 8.3. Tracing Each Element from the Center

6. Track and balance the energies.

A) Do the Divine Hook-Up: *Plug your left index finger into the heart of the Divine; use your right hand to bring Radiance into the conversation.*

Whether you are doing a quick or slow version of tracking your storyline, this is a key ingredient to clearing or resetting your templates. Radiance clears or opens the template for interaction and transformation. Usually, Radiance clears torqued and damaged energies fairly quickly. You might feel yourself take a deep breath, notice a settling in, or hear a kind of click of connection when it clears.

Continue to do this Divine Hook-Up the entire time you are in the space unless you need to use your hands for some kind of energy communication or to do an energy medicine exercise.

B) Explore what you find in this space. If you can turn off your thinking brain and treat this space like a dream space, you will probably find it easier to explore here. Where are you? What do you notice here? Who is here with you? Is anything happening? What is your sense of what the space needs: Does something need to be repaired, removed, transformed, rearranged, or added? Like in dreams, the storyline is often full of symbolic and metaphoric elements. You do not need to analyze these; you are just gathering impressions of what is there and what is needed. You may find yourself, like in a dream, engaged in some kind of interaction or task.

C) Call upon your Councils, kindred spirits in the World Wise Web, your Wiser Self, and/or the Universal Support Team to help you repair the space or rewrite the storyline. You may see immediately what is needed (e.g., a wall with holes in it, a car that has been taken apart and is all in pieces, or a flower that is wilting and needs to be watered). So feel free to step in and do what's needed. But don't feel you need to do all the work yourself—let your team help you do whatever you or they feel will bring this space into harmony.

D) Do energy medicine as needed to balance your energies where they live, relative to your inquiry. There are two basic ways to do this step if you choose to add it in. It is not necessary, but I find it is considerably more potent and effective to re-educate my energies when I am doing the exercise where the storyline lives.

The first way is to keep my attention in the chakra level space, and then just do the energy exercise as I would in general: a Third Eye–Belly Button Hook-Up (see page 38) or Porcupine Reset (see page 73) on my whole body.

The second way is to do these exercises in the space, in miniature. So, for example, I see myself (or a symbolic figure there) who is in reactivity, and I use my fingers to mime doing a Porcupine Reset or Coming Home on that little mini-me.

Basically, you can use any energy medicine technique or tool you've learned. The twist is that they will work a lot quicker, and go a lot deeper, when carried out in the context of Storyline Track and Balance.

When I am doing this technique, I ask myself, "What energy issue is going on here?" You can pose this question and just let your intuition suggest something that might help. But also, I have a quick checklist in my head. I look for:

◆ Gatekeeper reactivity

◆ Lack of grounding or orientation

◆ Blockage or lack of flow

◆ Evidence of electrical (nervous system) imbalance

◆ Structural issues (such as lack of supports, mushy containment)

◆ Lack of coordination, coherence, or things holding together

I'm providing you with a list of some possible energy medicine responses you could try if you sense need in one of these areas. Don't worry about getting the right exercise; you don't need to do *all* of these in any category, mostly one or two will suffice. Remember, energy medicine is also energy dialogue—if you try one, your body will respond and show you what it might need next. The deeper you are in a chakra, the faster these exercises work.

GATEKEEPER REACTIVITY

1. Porcupine Reset (page 73)

2. Pet the Doggy, Pet the Kitty (stroke behind ears like stroking your favorite pet)

3. Celtic Weave (page 93)

4. Consolation (either version) (pages 71, 80)

5. Clear Fear, Ease Ego, Welcome Wiser Self (page 37)

6. Coming Home (page 46)

7. Expanding Hearts (page 72)

8. Smart Filter (page 58)

GROUNDING OR ORIENTATION

1. Acrobat's Pole, Torus Pole, Yin-Yang Pole (page 119)

2. Hold the Storymaker anchors at feet, knees, Mingmen, heart, sides of face, sides of head (page 91)

3. Coming Home (page 46)

4. Reconciliation (page 8)

5. Third Eye–Belly Button Hook-Up (page 38)

6. Rabbit Ears (page 127)

7. Open angel wings on your scapula (Consolation, Version 2, Step 3) (page 80)

BLOCKAGE OR LACK OF FLOW

1. Celtic Clearing (page 105)

2. Celtic Weave (page 93)

3. Fascia massage: Self-massage to open skin by putting two fingers together on the skin, then stroking outward to stretch that area

4. Body Sweep (up front, down back) (page 56)

5. 3-5 Breathing (page 46)

6. Flip hand back and forth to clear polarities

7. Clear Frozen Eights (page 241)

ELECTRICAL (NERVOUS SYSTEM) IMBALANCE

1. Hold Storymaker anchors (page 91)

2. Do an *inner* Porcupine Reset, by starting and ending at the third eye instead of the top of the head.

3. Electrics Eye Hold: Hold closed eye lid and eyebrow bone at the same time.

4. Pet the Doggy, Pet the Kitty (stroke behind ears like stroking your favorite pet)

5. Do Coming Home (page 46)

6. Consolation (either version) (pages 71, 80)

7. Third Eye–Belly Button Hook-Up (page 38)

STRUCTURAL ISSUES

1. Harmonizing Hook-Up (page 195)

2. Trace shapes around your body or parts of your body (page 58)

3. Hold Storymaker anchors (page 91)

4. Trace a five-pointed star and circle over places that seem weak (page 110)

5. Adjust tailbone, reset face and nose (page 193)

6. Strengthen Body Weave (page 158)

7. Do the Basket Weave on your hand, focusing on the elements that need support (page 165)

COORDINATION, COHERENCE, THINGS HOLDING TOGETHER

1. Baklava Restoration (page 109)

2. Figure-eight and Celtic-weave between left and right sides of body (page 93)

3. Sing a scale up and down

4. Do Healing Hands, letting your hands show you where to connect (page 57)

5. Darn/re-weave any areas of the body that seem torn (page 156)

6. Do a Harmonizing Hook-Up (page 195)

7. Wrap yourself in a rainbow hammock or imagine yourself being held in a rainbow weave (page 195)

8. Open angel wings (page 80, Step 3)

7. When you feel that the energies are balanced at this level, trace the five-pointed star and circle to help seal the deal.

Starting with water and moving clock-wise, trace this star on your skin over the chakra you are traveling through. Imagine it printed there, with fire pointing up toward your head. When you place the star on your body this way, this reverses the image, so water element will be on your right side. (See Figure 8.4).

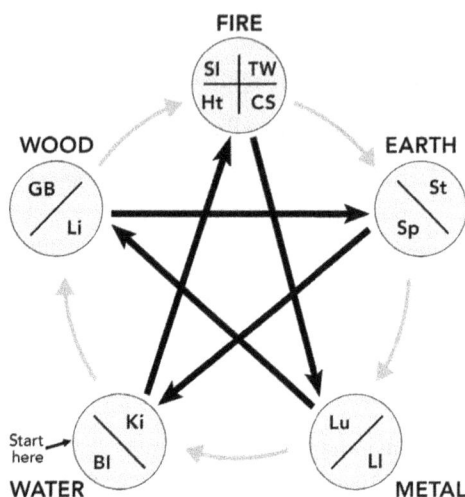

Figure 8.4. Trace the Five-Pointed Star and Circle, Starting with Water

8. Ask your guides for seeds of change to plant in the space.

Reach out your hand and ask your Councils or Wiser Self to give you the seeds of change that support your highest good. You do not need to specify which seeds you are asking for. Instead, let your Councils or Wiser Self gift you. Too often we try to plant what we *think* we want, rather than opening to our soul's input. And since what we think we want often relates to storylines that come from the socialized mind, it is good to let ourselves receive what the soul, spirit, and Wiser Self dimensions of our being have to offer.

9. Return to the surface to jot down or record what you experienced.

The communications and imagery you receive at each level are often like details in a dream. They can fade quickly. Therefore, I usually either return to the surface and jot down a few notes or use a voice recorder to capture what I want to remember.

Do you need to return to the surface each time? I have experimented with staying put and just voice recording my thoughts, and then dropping down to the next floor. For some people, returning to the surface helps them stay oriented and alert. It keeps them from losing track of where they are because, each time, they can count down which "floor" or level they are passing and which one they are on.

10. Proceed to the next level down in the same chakra, and repeat steps 4 to 9, using the same inquiry.

You do not need to track and balance all the layers of a chakra in a single session, though I often do. I find that as I travel through the layers, some balance quickly and others are juicier—filled with information and needing more attention. But, in general, the clearing gets quicker the deeper you go.

11. Review your notes to interpret what you've discovered.

After you've tracked the issue at all levels, you can spend some time figuring out what you've been shown. Remember that by bringing Radiance, you have already rebalanced the energies. Taking the time to interpret helps your mind catch up to what your energies are now doing. It isn't necessary, but it's often the most fun part!

As you review your notes to see what insights they give you, remember what each layer, each *place,* in your chakra represents. This allows you to interpret the details relative to what they refer to.

- ◆ **Level 1:** What is happening now in the **present story** of your life.

- ◆ **Level 2:** What is relevant to the present **phase of your life** (the past month or two or three).

- ◆ **Level 3:** What is relevant to the present **stage** of your life (the larger theme that may have been playing for several years).

- ◆ **Level 4:** Your **identity** in this life that you have built through positive and negative experience.

- ◆ **Level 5:** What **contracts or conditions** you set up to explore or express in this lifetime (including contracts to meet up and interact with others).

- **Level 6:** What **past life or counterpart life events** are coloring your story (bleed-through from past lives).

- **Level 7:** What **cosmic influences** are influencing your field (including bleed-through from other dimensions of reality and larger astrological tides).

Guided Visit: Storyline Track and Balance

To get the most out of the guided visits in this book, you can either record the text for yourself, leaving silent spaces to allow yourself to explore as guided, or you can download an MP3 recording I've provided and use that. See page 13 for instructions on how to access the MP3s.

If you are using the downloadable MP3 recording, it includes guidance for each of these levels. If you are creating your own recording, you can just reread the level-specific instructions and substitute the correct level name each time. In the MP3, where energy exercises are suggested, you can substitute any you find in the chart on pages 220–221, or any others that you feel will address the imbalance you perceive.

Before you start your visit, take a few moments to identify what issue or storyline you want to track. Find a simple phrase to represent it through this journey (e.g., "This situation with my mother" or "Getting headaches from strawberries").

As a preliminary exercise, we're going to start with Porcupine Reset. With both hands, grasp your energy at the top of your head. Inhale and pull upward to arm's length. As you exhale, bring your hands, still clutching the energy, down in an arc as if you are a big egg and you are tracing the shell. Pull the energy all the way to the floor (as close as you can reach) and tack it down.

Now, grasp the energy at the bottom of your egg, inhale, and pull it upward, bowing out along your egg shape, and tack it at the top of your head on the exhale.

Now, calm any inner porcupine reactivity. Moving your hands to your third eye, on your forehead, grasp the energy there, inhale, and pull the energies up, outward, then bowing out and down along your eggshell shape. On the exhale, tack them to the ground.

Inhale, and grasping the energies from the bottom of your egg, pull them up, bowing outward along your eggshell, and on the exhale, tack them back to your third eye.

Take three deep breaths in through your nose and out through your mouth. Trace hearts on your heart area as you do this deep breathing.

Now, ask your chakras, "Show me the priority chakra to track templates for *[name your issue]*." Place a hand on each chakra in turn to see where you feel the strongest pull or feel your hand sink in. If you want, you can ask the priority chakra to light up in your mind's eye, or let your hand just fall intuitively where you can most fruitfully track your story.

Keep breathing in through your nose and out through your mouth. If a priority chakra does not signal to you, just use your intuition to choose one. You can't do this wrong.

Place your hand on the chosen chakra, and say, "Looking for templates relating to *[add your phrase]*." Feel your hand there on the chakra, and ask for a passageway to open between the surface and the first level down. It might show up as a door, a tunnel, an opening, or you might wish to just use an elevator or escalator to travel down to the first level.

Once you are there, using a star shape on the surface of the chakra where you started, trace each arm of the five-element star to open the conversation. Start at the center of the star, and trace outward to the bottom right side, where water sits. Tune in to see if this connection feels strong or challenged, and anything else about it that comes to mind.

Then return to the center of the star, and trace outward to the middle right side of the star, where wood sits. Again, tune in to whatever you pick up about this connection.

Return to the center of the star, and trace upward to the top of the star, fire. What does that connection feel like?

Return to the center of the star again, and this time, trace to the left, feeling into the center-to-earth connection.

And, finally, from the center of the star, trace down and to the left to take a sounding of the center-to-metal connection.

Breathe in through your nose and out through your mouth, keeping your attention in the first layer of your chakra and feeling the five arms of the star you have just drawn.

Now, you are going to bring Radiance in using a Divine Hook-Up. Plug your left index finger into the heart of the Divine or whatever you hold sacred. If your arm is extended in the air, invite the Divine to squat down, so you are not in an uncomfortable position! Feel the Radiance from the Source you are plugged into traveling down your arm and throughout your Yin-Yang axis, emanating out your right hand and fingers.

Use that Radiance to fill the chakra space you find yourself in. You are merely a conduit for this Radiance. You do not need to direct it or even make it flow. Just open to it, and let its intelligence find the correct distribution.

Explore with your mind this layer of the chakra. What do you notice about the space you are in? What do you feel here? Are you alone, or are there others here? Are you part of the scene or just observing?

Let the place speak to you; let it show you what is needed and what is going on with the storyline here. Just note as much as you can, and if there is no detail, inhabit the space and continue to hold the Divine Hook-Up, letting it do its magic.

If you wish, invite your guides or Councils to join you in this space. Ask the Universal Support Team to bring in whatever is needed: supplies, replacement parts, free labor, and the like. The intelligence of the Radiance and your helpers, plus your own insights, can guide whatever needs to happen to make this space what it needs to be right now.

Also tune in to your own energies or the energies of the selves you find in the space. Do they need help to get their energies flowing? If you're not sure, quickly do one of the exercises I'm about to mention, depending on your needs:

+ Do you need to help calm reactivity? If so, try doing a Porcupine Reset on your whole self or on your mini-me in that space, and trace hearts on your heart.

+ If you need help with grounding, hold a few Storymaker anchors, perhaps the knees and sides of the face.

+ If there is blockage, do a Body Sweep from your feet up the front of your body to the top of your head, and from your shoulders, out along the insides of your arms to your fingertips. Then sweep down the backs of your arms from your fingertips to your neck, and next sweep the energy from your crown down your back and off the sides of your feet.

+ If there is nervous system imbalance, do the Electrics Eye Hold, holding your closed eye lid together with the bony surround of your eye. Place one finger on your closed eyelid and the other on the bone you feel under your eyebrow.

+ If your structures seem wonky, do a Harmonizing Hook-Up, with one hand on the front of your left shoulder and the other on the front of your left pelvis, and imagine yourself being rocked in a rainbow hammock.

+ And if you feel a lack of coherence, sing a scale up and down.

When you feel that this space is balanced or your work is complete, trace a five-pointed star and circle to seal the deal. Hold out your palm to receive seeds of change from your Wiser Self or Councils. When you feel the seeds in your palm, bring them into the space and plant them. Water them, throw in a little organic "Miracle Grow," thank your guides and helpers, and using your breath, bring your attention back to the surface with your exhale.

Take a moment to jot down or voice record everything you experienced in the space.

When you are ready, repeat your intention: "Looking for templates related to [name your issue]." Look for a passage or get in your elevator to travel down to the second level. Trace each arm of the five-pointed star from the center outward, starting with center—water. Explore the space to see what is going on and what is needed here. Do the Divine Hook-Up to bring in Radiance. Call in helpers and guides to help with whatever is needed. And check in with your body to see what energy medicine exercises would be helpful to you in this space.

When the space feels complete, trace the five-pointed star and circle, thank your helpers, ask for seeds of change for your highest good, and plant them in the newly renovated space. Water and fertilize them, and then use your exhales to return your awareness to the surface.

Take a moment to jot down or voice record everything you experienced in the space.

Repeat this process for the third, fourth, fifth, sixth, and seventh levels of the chakra.

When you are finished, trace a five-pointed star and circle on the surface to seal the deal.

●　●　●

Take your time interpreting what you've discovered. The storyline you were tracking will be balanced but may well lead you to recognize other storylines that need some revision.

Janice noticed something strange happening to her. Every time she had a conversation that lasted more than ten minutes with her mother, she developed a bladder infection within an hour. "The strange thing is," she said, "it isn't really stress. I love my mother, in some ways she's my closest friend." The bladder infections had started four years ago, within weeks of Janice getting married, but clearly only came up when she engaged with her mother. It was driving her crazy and starting to hurt her mother's feelings. Janice was worried that all the antibiotics would cause other damage and wanted to know if energy medicine could help.

It is just the kind of mystery that Storyline Track and Balance is good for. The day she came to see me, she had a raging UTI. We talked about whether to track the storyline identifier: "This situation with my mother" or to use "These bladder infections." Since the infections seemed most urgent, we decided to start there.

The storyline showed up in her first, second, third, fourth, and fifth chakras when we tested them, meaning it was a big deal, woven through much of her being. The priority chakra was not her first or second chakras, which are physically closest to her bladder. It was her heart chakra.

On the first level down, present situation, she was "blotto" (meaning her control and flow cycles were not working). We brought Radiance, and she said that it looked like she had come apart. That she was just a pile of parts, like a Picasso painting. She called in the Universal Support Team to reassemble her, and she sang a musical scale up and down to re-establish coherence.

On the second level down, this phase of her life, her water element was out of balance, but the others tested strong. She saw herself rowing in a boat that had a hole in it. She was trying to get to an island that she said was called "Saint's Island" but had to keep stopping to bail out the boat, and so she wasn't getting anywhere. The Universal Support Team offered her a choice: Repair this boat or swap it for a fancier motorboat. She decided it felt like cheating to use a motorboat to get to Saint's Island. It seemed to her that it was important to get there under her own steam. They repaired the boat, and I did a Harmonizing Hook-Up for her while she held hands with the Divine. (This is the advantage of working with a helper—they can do some of the energy medicine while you bring Radiance.)

At the third level, the present stage of her life, she was in a fog. She couldn't see anything. The fog was not threatening or scary. But she said, "I'm just being held in place by it. I don't dare move because I don't know what's there." She did Coming Home to calm the part of her that wanted to freak out in the fog. Bringing the Radiance gradually helped to move the fog out. And, as it did, she found herself in an amazing greenhouse filled with plants. There were gorgeous flowering plants, herbs, thistles, and succulents, all growing in there together and thriving. She said, "I'm the head gardener here, but I forgot it even existed!" She asked her Councils to send her a staff to help take care of the place and laughed when she planted seeds: "I'm curious," she said, "what they could possibly add to this place!"

On the fourth level, representing her identity, she found herself in a kind of sports competition. She was in a tug-of-war, and her mother and husband were both on her team, pulling against another team she couldn't see. It was taking all her strength to just hold against that force pulling against them. I asked her what she wanted to have happen there. She said, "I'd like to get out of this competition, but since I don't know who's at the other end of the rope, I'm afraid to just let go." She decided to ask the Universal Support Team to send in substitutes so that she and her mother and husband could release the rope. She also asked for a referee to make decisions about the contest, so she wouldn't worry. We reset her Acrobat's Pole, Torus Pole, and Yin-Yang Pole, because she felt the contest had somehow pulled her seriously out of balance. We ended with a Celtic Weave to shift her energies from tugging to integration.

On the fifth level, representing contracts and conditions she set on this life, she and her mother were sitting and whispering together and giggling. She said, "I can't hear what we are saying, but it's so sweet. I just want to hang out and be silly with her." She had a strong emotional reaction and started to cry. I invited her to do Expanding Hearts and call in both of their Wiser Selves. She invited her Wiser Self to stand behind her, and her mother's Wiser Self to stand behind her mother, so they were each being supported. The scene faded, and she saw herself in another moment from her college years. It was the night she had decided to lose her virginity. She said, "I was both mad at myself and pleased to finally have taken the plunge. I didn't particularly enjoy it, and the guy wasn't someone I wanted to be in a relationship with. And, because of that, I felt I couldn't tell my mom. I didn't want her to be disappointed in me." I asked her what she wanted to see happen. She decided to figure-eight between her and her mom and to trace figure eights over her root chakra to reclaim it as hers.

On the sixth level, representing past lives or counterpart-self events, she found herself in a house of sorrow, as she put it. There was a mother, father, and a little kid. She realized she was the little kid in the scene, and she was heartbroken. Her older sister had just been *given* in marriage to a much older man. She did not want to go. The mother and father were not showing any emotion; they were just working and looking grim.

"Do you know who her sister was?" I asked. She replied, "My mom in this life. She was my best friend then too."

I asked her what was needed. . . .

She said, "I'm not sure. I want to know what happened to her."

I asked her if she wanted to look, and she said, "No, I'm too scared. Can my guides just tell me?" She called in her Councils and asked them what happened to that older sister. They were kind and loving and said, "She never adjusted to her new home. She did not love her husband and ended up dying in childbirth a few years later. You were more fortunate: You married a man from the church you quite liked and lived into your fifties, relatively contented."

Janice wasn't sure what to do for her mother and for herself. She decided to Celtic-weave her mother and then hold her own Storymaker anchors. This story made her feel unmoored and guilty. Holding the anchors calmed that guilt. She then sent hearts to each character in that storyline.

On the seventh level, the level of cosmic influence, all was calm, and the five-pointed star was strong and intact. So she spent a few seconds bringing Radiance, and then traced a five-pointed star and circle, and returned her consciousness to the surface.

And she discovered, when she excused herself to go to the bathroom, her bladder infection was gone—no pain, no inflammation, and no itch.

What Janice was shown in this process was not just a pat answer to what was happening ("Oh, it was a past life drama with your mother"), but instead she saw the interplay of elements in her life, in her relationships, and in her makeup that were co-creating the storyline. And, by tracking it using Radiance, the symbolic language of energy, and energy medicine, she was able to transform and balance the templates and shift her body's response to it.

I heard from Janice a few years later, saying she had stopped having bladder infections, but she also wanted me to know that her relationship with her mother had shifted too. They were still very close, but each of them now felt they were better at both being close and giving each other space. Janice also reported that her marriage was fine, with normal ups and downs, but greatly benefiting from her being available for intimacy without all the UTIs.*

COUNTERPART SELVES AND MULTI-DIMENSIONAL HEALING

Storyline Track and Balance does not have to be used only when there is a problem or illness. It can be used to bring Radiance to any storyline and glean insights about it. At the sixth level of her chakra, Janice dropped into what seemed like a past-life memory. It gave her insights about her present relationship with her mother and also gave her a chance to do some healing work for the little girl and sister who she felt were counterparts to her and her mother.

One aspect of multi-dimensional healing is to get to know the selves you have been in other lives—and the counterpart selves who relate to you in some way now. Over the years, my Councils have taken me to meet many of my past selves, in part to illuminate issues I was having in my present life. I don't subscribe to the belief that our problems in this life are *caused* by past lives. But I do think the soul explores key issues in multiple settings. So, if your soul is exploring loss and gain, you'll have a whole slew of lifetimes where this theme is playing out. My Councils described it like leaves on a bush. Each of these lifetimes are like leaves that face the sun in their own way and feed the whole bush. Since we are oriented to the timeline, we think

---

* Not all Storyline Track and Balance sessions end with the physical symptoms gone and emotional and energetic issues resolved. That is partly because many challenges reflect multiple storylines, and/or sometimes you may need more than one visit to balance all the templates. Also sometimes, after clearing the energetic source of a physical problem, the body may still need additional time and energy medicine support to heal.

in terms of past and future lives. But I love to just see it as your counterpart selves on the bush.

One fun way to use Storyline Track and Balance is to track the connections you have with another person through all the levels of your chakras to learn about various aspects of how your lives are intertwined. When you get to the sixth level down, which is a particularly rich place to meet your past and counterpart selves, you can learn about your other-life connections to the person you are tracking. You can also, when tracking a particular issue, make sure at the sixth level to ask what other lives you've lived that explored that issue.

|||||||||||||| **Play with It!** ||||||||||||||

Ask for insight about how a certain relationship or core theme plays out in your life. Do a Storyline Track and Balance down through the levels to get insight into how this issue shows up in your lived experience (the first three levels), in your identity and construction of self (the fourth level), in the contracts you set up as a soul coming into this life (the fifth level), in the counterpart lives you've lived (sixth level), and in the cosmic dimensions (seventh level).

Spend some extra time at the sixth level, asking your guides to show you past or counterpart selves that relate to the theme/issue or person you are tracking. Or ask a past-life self to show up there, and tell you their story. Do not worry if these past lives are real! You'll find that out after this lifetime. Treat the characters you get to know as maps of understanding that can deepen your sense of who you are and have been.

Often you will get a good sense of what some of the key issues, or cutting edge of growth, were in each of your lives, rather than details about identity in the world. And, really, your identity was just a costume your soul put on in that life. Let the essence of the various parts of yourself show itself to you as you visit that space.

●　●　●

Tracking your storylines, bringing the communications and energy conversations to where they live, allows you to awaken to how rich and multi-dimensional you truly are. It helps you expand your limited sense of self and bring Radiance to all parts of your being.

In chapter 9, we'll explore another rich territory of your multi-dimensional self—the Field of Possibility.

CHAPTER NINE

Playing in Your Field of Possibility

Sonya was one of those people who seem to have a KICK ME sign on her. She got flagged and sent to me by an energy medicine teacher-in-training who wondered if Sonya had "entities" attached to her somehow. Everywhere this beleaguered soul went, things would start to get chaotic. It wasn't any overt behavior on her part: Sonya was mostly quiet and respectful. But when she was in the room, the teacher said, her classmates all started to avoid her and lose their focus or just feel bad. The teacher finally asked her to leave the class until she could get her energies balanced. She sent her to me, asking if I could clear the entities. "Even my dog couldn't stand to have her around," she told me.

My heart went out to Sonya. She didn't have entities attached to her in the sense her teacher meant. Because of my woo-woo training, I was occasionally asked by colleagues to consult on situations that looked like they involved entities. They almost never did. Instead, Sonya had what I have come to think of as a booby-trapped Gatekeeper. And she had templates in her chakras and energy artifacts in her Field of Possibility that created chaos around her.

In fact, one-on-one, Sonya was quite sweet. And it hurt her deeply that this had happened, though she didn't blame the teacher-in-training, because it was what Sonya experienced nearly every time she tried to participate in some group activity. I asked her to tell me her story.

Sonya was Croatian and grew up in Bosnia during the Bosnian War. Her family, like most families there, was repeatedly traumatized not just by the violence and fear but by the betrayals of people they thought were friends, neighbors, allies. She grew up with constant warnings that she must be vigilant, both socially and physically, because of the land mines. A neighbor kid she played with before the war lost his leg when he kicked a stone that turned out not to be a stone.

"We were lucky," she said. "My mother had a sister who had emigrated to the States years earlier. She was able to get us out and bring us over here." Sonya was about ten years old at the time. At first, she was so happy to be free of the stresses of war that she just dove into her American experience headfirst. She learned English in a few months and spoke it with very little accent. She made friends, worked hard in school, and basically felt she had landed in paradise.

But after a few years, she started to feel unsafe again. Classmates would turn on her, for no apparent reason, or exclude her from parties everyone else was invited to. Several teachers told her that she needed therapy. But they couldn't (or wouldn't) tell her why. Her parents, worried about her mental health, sent her to a therapist, who helped her process her traumatic past and gave her some skills to cope with the disruptions she was experiencing. That helped her get through college, feeling more or less okay. She was not particularly popular—she was by then a bit of a loner—but she wasn't actively ostracized.

After graduating, she started a mail-order business that did not require her to be in an office, exposed to the sometimes-fraught group dynamics. But she always felt something was wrong with her. Too many friendships ended with a sense of betrayal or unfair rejection. Too many times, she had joined a group, only to get kicked out. She had signed up for the energy medicine class, hoping to understand her energies better and break this pattern, only to run into it once again.

Like the land-mined territory Sonya had to navigate as a child, her multidimensional self had at first been protected by energy templates, telling her Gatekeeper how to keep her safe. But over time, these same safeguards became obstacles, blocking Sonya from moving forward.

A booby-trapped Gatekeeper is a Gatekeeper that has set up protections that are so strong you can't just override them and turn them off. It is an autopilot that runs away with the ship. It is a lockbox that requires a combination you no longer remember. It is a field full of mines that presents an ongoing danger because you don't have a map for where the mines got planted.

This can take many forms. You might have templates that just shut people out automatically, repel them in some way, or close you down without giving you a chance to decide on a case-by-case basis. This was happening to Sonya. Or your Gatekeeper might have templates, like a KICK ME sign, that repeatedly call in situations that re-traumatize you, perhaps in a misguided attempt by your Gatekeeper to give your Storymaker a chance to write new templates. This was also happening to Sonya, whose Gatekeeper had booby-trapped her ability to enjoy membership in groups and wasn't letting her Storymaker write new stories.

Once some aspect of your energies has been designated as a danger zone (or some other kind of fixed zone), your Gatekeeper can, on the one hand, shut your energies down, freeze them, or block them, so you can't enter what it has designated as a threat. On the other hand, it can make your energies too open, put you into overdrive, but unable to learn, so you can't leave the danger zone behind. People with love addictions or manic tendencies, or who chronically somatize experiences in their bodies without feeling them emotionally, often have Gatekeepers who have booby-trapped their gates-of-self to stay too wide open.

Sonya knew she carried a belief that life is not safe, that she was not safe. She had tried energy tapping to clear that belief and tried using affirmations to shift her fear. These techniques had helped some, but her Gatekeeper wasn't buying it. It was as if something in her was so cracked or so miswired that her Gatekeeper was not going to be sweet-talked into giving up its booby traps.

I want to be clear here: In many situations, energy tapping, which involves invoking a situation and tapping certain acupuncture points to balance your energies relative to that situation, can be very effective, even miraculous. But since it involves clearing trauma via the meridian streams, it doesn't always reach to all the dimensions of the self—for example, into the chakras or out into the Field of Possibility or into the master template I call your harmonic self.

And belief work is great for schooling your Storymaker to create new beliefs. After all, beliefs help shape the templates of experience your Storymaker creates. But belief work doesn't necessarily clear energy templates, which as you may have already discovered, can be amazingly tenacious.

That's why I advocate going beyond the concepts of *clearing trauma* or *programming yourself to change*, to instead work on *transforming trauma and templates of experience where they live*, in partnership with your Storymaker and Gatekeeper.

And that's how we helped Sonya un-booby-trap her energies. She did a number of Storyline Track and Balance sessions to encounter and bring Radiance to the templates from her past experiences, transforming them to templates that affirmed her soul's truth and helped her Gatekeeper find safety.

She also worked with her Storymaker's anchoring, framing, weaving, sourcing, and steering mechanisms, as I've described throughout this book. She basically made new configurations in her inner workings that gave her Gatekeeper better instructions on how to keep the gates of self. Once she (and her Storymaker) were rewoven within, her Gatekeeper could relax a bit.

However, because much of the trauma Sonya had suffered came from *out there*, from the Web of Connections, from the world she was living in, and from physical danger that was beyond her personal ability to protect herself, she also needed to heal and transform some additional places within her multi-dimensional self—in particular, her Field of Possibility and her harmonic self. Basically, these are energies that allow us to create our reality and to call in experiences via the Web of Connections. Keep reading—I'll explain what this all means and give you some tools that help you work with it yourself.

YOUR FIELD OF POSSIBILITY

I like to think of the Field of Possibility as your drawing board—as in "let's go back to the drawing board." It's an energetic workspace where your Storymaker can craft stories and set up plans, intentions, sample frameworks, and tentative maps of experience. It's where we try experiences on for size and shape our intentions and choices. And it's a rich place to use your imagination to expand your potential.

Your Field of Possibility starts at your energetic core, extends outward encompassing your aura, and even extends a bit beyond, overlapping with the energies that come to you via the Web of Connections—the weave that links us to other people and the world around us. When a clairvoyant sees illnesses approaching you in your aura or sees disturbances coming into your sphere to color your aura, they are probably seeing the stories your Storymaker is investigating, starting to frame, or drafting in its workspace—the Field of Possibility. (See Figure 9.1.)

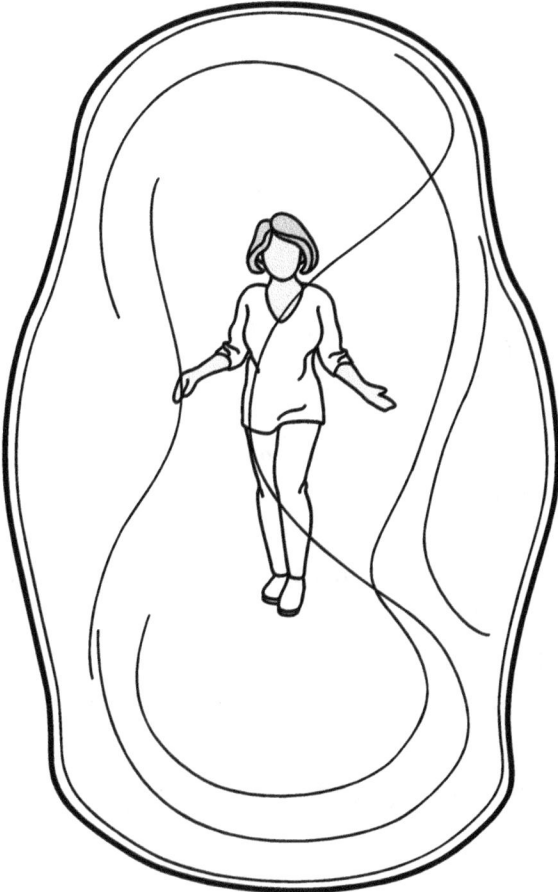

Figure 9.1. The Field of Possibility

We are more familiar in our shared culture with the concept of *aura*, the magnetic field surrounding your body that acts like the atmosphere protecting our planet. It is fed by your chakras, and like all subtle energies, it is ultimately part of your consciousness and carries meaning. It acts as an interface between your world *in there* and your world *out there*, and sometimes, as in Sonya's case, it is cluttered with so much pollution and distortion that it can impede the health of your body.

Your Field of Possibility encompasses and influences your aura (and vice versa), but your Field of Possibility is larger and more dimensional, somehow. It gives you access to the whole spectrum of who you are and can be: your multi-dimensional self.

Sonya's Gatekeeper had booby-trapped her Field of Possibility to keep her safe. It kept her in a small, unimaginative life with very little ability to truly prosper as a soul having a human experience. It also kept her from cultivating and planting seeds in this field—to create a reality her heart and imagination yearned for.

> *Reality isn't a fixed thing—it is a composite of what might be, is, and has been. It is a composite of lived and imagined and projected experiences.*

> *By the same token, your Experience isn't a fixed thing—it is a complex of moving, shifting, energetic forces that morph all over the place. It is a composite of memory, perception, action, and codified understanding.*

Both reality and experience are more spectrum-y, more nuanced, more dimensional than we usually recognize in our culture. That's why we can interact with our energies at various places in our multi-dimensional self and heal, bring in new possibilities, and create new patterns for the body and mind.

BRAKES, BAFFLES, AND GATING

I have various names for the Gatekeeper artifacts and pollution that kept Sonya in a locked box: *brakes, baffles, gating, frozen energies, irregular energies,* and more. Clearing templates in her chakras helped her stop trashing her energy field. Getting her Storymaker working better also helped clean up her energies. But just as we need to clean up all kinds of detritus trashing our yard after a big storm, we can also have energy artifacts littering our subtle energies.

The exercise on page 105, Celtic Clearing, is an excellent way to sweep out some of the crap that has invaded your Field of Possibility. But, sometimes, when you go to sweep, things don't clear. Then it's good to look for brakes, baffles, and gating.

Brakes

Brakes are basically energies that have frozen or stopped moving the way they need to move. If you are scanning your energies with your hands, you might experience them as a place where energy is cold, not moving, or feels stuck. Since energies are meant to move, energies that are blocked, in stasis, or diverted from their flow will act as brakes for your Storymaker, stopping forward motion in your creation of self. In some ways, it is an effective protection to stop poisons (emotional, physical, and energetic) from spreading. But, although they protect us, brakes in the movements of our energies also degrade our health.

Exercise: Clear Frozen Eights

Our subtle energies travel in figure-eight patterns. Donna Eden has frequently commented that the more figure eights she sees in someone's energy field, the healthier they tend to be.

A frozen eight is a figure-eight pattern that is sluggish or barely moving. It is an artifact of the Gatekeeper that puts an electromagnetic "freeze" on energy movement as a form of self-protection. This is part of our flight, fight, or freeze reactivity. When we have a frozen eight, the energy communications in that area are greatly slowed down or impeded. This is self-protective but annoying, like many immune system reactions! It also pretty much locks out most energy techniques and conversations.

You can learn to feel for frozen eights. Rub your hands together to activate the energies there. Then, with your palm facing your body, about two to three inches above the surface, scan for places that feel still, cold, and/or less energized somehow. You can bring in your imagination, seeing in your mind's eye which areas are red and warm, and which are cold and white or blue. Or listen for the sounds of movement versus stillness. Or just let direct knowing tell you, "There's a frozen eight here."

Since the figure eights of our energies flow every which way and are big and small, you can also scan your aura, send your sensors down into your body and into your organs, and even scan your Field of Possibility for frozen or stuck energies.

If you wish to energy test for frozen eights, place your hands at either end of where you believe a frozen eight sits (see Figure 9.2). Then energy test: A weak test indicates you have found a frozen eight (see Appendix A for some simple energy test instructions). You can also, in this case, use a pendulum and scan your body and field. When it encounters a frozen eight, your pendulum will generally slow down or stop moving.

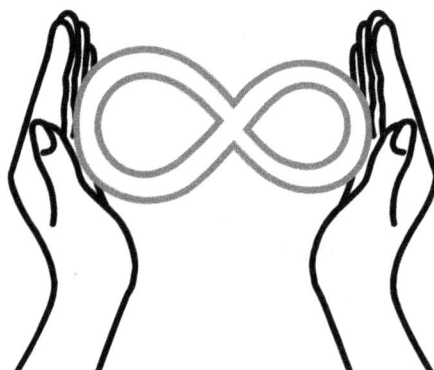

Figure 9.2. Figure Eight Between Hands

Frozen eights can often be found around key functions: crossing the heart, crossing the brain, from top to bottom of your whole body, across the gut, and so forth. Wherever function is impeded, you can check to see if there is a frozen eight in the field.

To correct a frozen eight:

1. Place your hands at either end of where you perceive/imagine the eight to be and then slowly push the palms of your hands toward each other, squashing the eight between them (see Figure 9.3a).

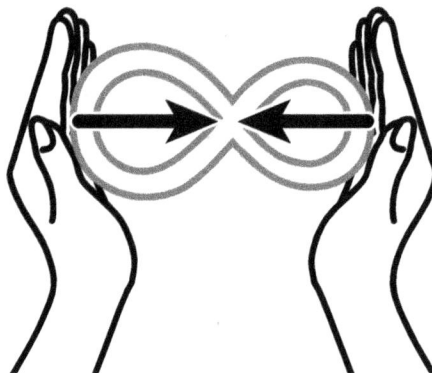

Figure 9.3a. Squashing the Eight

2. Once your palms meet (in the prayer position), place your hands back to back and continue pushing outward with each hand (arms now crossed) toward the edges of where you imagine or perceive the eight sits (see Figure 9.3b).

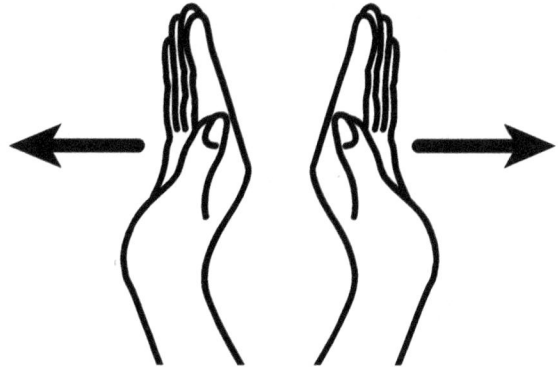

Figure 9.3b. Pushing to the Edges of the Eight

3. After you have cleared the frozen eight, figure-eight in the same area to reanimate good flow.

It is sometimes useful to be able to sense where the eights are, and for that reason, I have taught you how to locate and test for them. But, if you prefer, you can do what Sonya chose, which was to clear her eights, every which way, once a day. She basically did the eight-squashing correction from head to foot, left to right, front to back, at angles in her body, and every which way in her aura to just clear out the freeze that had accumulated there from so many years of Gatekeeper lockdown.

Baffles

According to *Merriam-Webster*, a "baffle" is "a device (such as a plate, wall, or screen) to deflect, check, or regulate flow or passage (as of a fluid, light, or sound)." Or, I might add, subtle energy. Baffles get set up like dams in our energies to allow Gatekeeper to block flow, cutting off circulation. It may seem self-defeating, but a baffle acts as a circuit breaker, allowing the Gatekeeper to control and ration energies when, for some reason, it thinks resources won't be renewed.

To me, baffles look a little like a wall or partition. I often find them cutting off a body part, separating top from bottom, or in any place where something has been disowned by my client (or myself) or people around them. For example, someone with unusually fat legs might have baffles between their torso and thigh, someone whose head and heart don't communicate well might have a baffle at the base or top of their neck, or someone who has a bad knee might have a baffle just below or above it. It is the crazy logic of the Gatekeeper, trying to keep the area from getting overwhelmed but, in the process, also cutting off necessary energetic and even physiological flow. An energetic baffle can impede blood, nourishment, and nerve messaging from getting to an area.

We are familiar with the concept of baffles in emotional terms: We'll say something like "He lives a compartmentalized life," or "She has partitioned her feelings because they were too overwhelming for her." In energetic terms, I'd say, "They have baffles." And baffles, being an energetic feature, can be cleared.

Exercise: Clearing Baffles

Before clearing baffles, it is useful to calm your Gatekeeper by doing the Porcupine Reset (see page 73) and drawing hearts on your heart. This minimizes any potential reactivity on the part of your Gatekeeper to having you mess with its controls!

Baffles can usually be found near energy blockage, or wherever you have a sense of separation in your body or energy field, including your Field of Possibility. In your body, you will probably be able to intuit where they are, because they sit between places where energy seems to be flowing and energy is not working well.

In your aura and in your Field of Possibility, they exist in places where energies coming in or going out were overwhelming your Gatekeeper. Often, they get set up to block access from the world to your heart, eyes, ears, nose, brain, or feet. Unfortunately, while cutting off flow inward from the world, they also impede your ability to express yourself outward.

Many people can feel baffles. Sweep your hand slowly through your field, perhaps emphasizing the areas where you might take energies in from the world. For example, with your palm facing outward, start at your face and slowly move your hand outward. If there is a baffle there, it will feel like a slight impediment, a bit of resistance.

If you have learned any energy tests, you can do a polarity test there: With your palm facing the baffle, energy test. It should test strong. With your hand facing away from the baffle, energy test. It should test weak. Any other configuration means there is a baffle there. (See Appendix A for more on energy testing.)

But you don't need to energy test if you don't want to. Clearing a baffle that isn't there does no harm.

To clear the baffle, imagine it is a circuit breaker, and turn it off and then on again, the way you would flip the switch on an actual circuit breaker. I usually flip it right to left, then left to right. But however you imagine it works fine.

Then, use a Divine Hook-Up (see page 37) to bring Radiance and clear the baffle. If you tune in to it while you bring Radiance, you may be able to get it to "talk" to you and to show you when and why it got set up.

If a baffle is serving an important purpose now, rather than being an artifact from past storms, then don't worry—your Gatekeeper will replace it rapidly. Then your mission is to address that purpose in another way. For example, if you have an intrusive relative, the baffle may serve as a protection. Your job would then be to find another way to fortify yourself when around that person.

Gating

In a way, baffles are a form of gating. They are set up to block traffic in an area. A more advanced form of gating is when your Gatekeeper decides to box or lock an area in. In other words, instead of a single baffle standing between you and your sore lower back, you might find a four- or six-sided energetic box there, protecting the area in its vulnerability—and, unfortunately, protecting it in many cases from getting better.

If you have a part of your body or mind that is chronically in pain, out of balance, challenged, or not healing properly, there's a good chance there is also some gating there. Sonya had gating around her entire body. Her Gatekeeper had just set her into a protective box, labeled "no entry," and while it allowed some energies to get to her, it also clearly sent the message to all who met her to beware and back off. She also had boxes around her heart and her head.

Once we cleared her gating, she experienced an immediate shift in how people reacted to her. She said it was as if she had been wrapped in cotton most of her life, and now she could feel the world around her again.

It is fairly easy to locate and correct gating. However, work with gating can also lead into very deep, nuanced dialogue with one's Gatekeeper and Storymaker, and it can help you clear body memories and habit templates stored in the body. Therefore, I usually treat this technique as a conversation with my Storymaker and Gatekeeper, and I use it to investigate how my story got codified in this stuck way. The gating can also indicate when (in this and other lifetimes) this issue was so strong that it needed to be gated. It can often yield insights into the stories that caused your Gatekeeper to create it. Like clearing templates using Storyline Track and Balance, I've seen people have *miracle* releases and healing after clearing a gated area of their body or mind or Field of Possibility.

Protocol: Clear Gatekeeper Gating

Note: This protocol can be quite an advanced practice or can be used simply to remove electromagnetic artifacts. If it feels too complicated to you to use it to get information, just focus on the action of locating, unlocking, unlatching, and dissolving each side of the box. Having said that, I'm a big advocate of asking for insight when interacting with energies and letting them speak to me. Most of us are more capable of that than we think!

This protocol begins much like the exercise to clear baffles. As a preliminary step, do the Porcupine Reset (see page 73) to calm your yang Gatekeeper, protecting you from the world *out there.* And trace hearts on your heart to calm your yin Gatekeeper, protecting the inner sanctity of your *self.*

1. Locate the gating.

You can use your intuition to find the gating, like with feeling for baffles. Scan with your hand to feel for one of the "walls" of an energy box or ask the side of the box to show up on your mental screen. As mentioned, the difference between a baffle and gating is that a baffle is generally just a single partition. Gating is usually something that puts the area in a protective/restrictive box. When an area is boxed, it might have baffles on two, four, or six sides. I don't recall ever encountering gating on one side of a gated area that wasn't bracketed on the other side.

2. See if the box is electromagnetically locked.

Skip this step if you are using your intuition to give you information about the box. If you wish to energy test, use the polarity test I described previously (see page 245). The palm of the hand facing the area being protected should test strong; the palm of the hand facing away from the protected area should test weak. Since it is a box, the orientation of strong is always toward the box, and weak is always away from the box.

3. Unlock the box.

If you sense or discover via energy test that the gate is "locked," meaning its energetic polarity has flipped and is not allowing energy to flow, release this lock by grasping the side of the box you are working with top and bottom, inhale, and on the exhale, flip it like a Frisbee, so the side formerly facing outward now faces inward.

Note: At this point in the book, I imagine you are aware that when I say, "Grasp the side of the box," I mean, use gesture to mime the action, as a way of communicating to the energies what you are asking them to do.

4. Unlatch the latches.

Most gated boxes are both locked electromagnetically and latched shut. This makes it difficult to shift them. There may be one or multiple energetic "latches" holding the gate (and associated reactivity) in place. Use your intuition and feel along the side of your box you are working on for latches.

Usually, the latches are on the right side, the way they would be on a door. But I have worked with gating where the latches were on the top (hatch-door style) or bottom or left side as well. Since energy is nonlocal, don't sweat if you don't know exactly where the latches are. Your intention will create the link that allows you to communicate "opening" to the latch.

To feel or test for a latch, crook your index finger and place the side of the crooked finger on the spot where you suspect a latch (often on the left or right edge of the gate). If you are using intuition, you will just sense *Here's a latch.* If you are energy testing, place this crooked finger along the edge of the box where you think the latch is and energy test (see Figure 9.4). A weak test shows you have found a latch.*

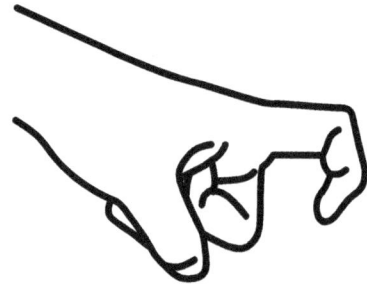

Figure 9.4.
Energy Test for a Latch

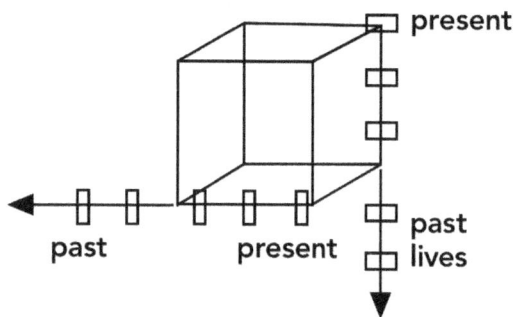

Figure 9.5. Gating and the Timeline

Often you can tell *when*, in this life or another, the latch was set up and what the circumstances were. Each edge of the box can act as a kind of timeline, a geological record of when the events happened that created this box (see Figure 9.5).

Starting at the top edge of the side with the latches (on vertical planes) or the front edge of the side with the latches (on horizontal planes), that corner is the present time. The first latch might be halfway along that edge, meaning it got set up midway through your life to date. Another latch might be lower on the edge, indicating childhood, or on the bottom corner, meaning at or before birth. If

---

* For more experienced energy testers: To make sure you are not just energy localizing a weak spot, you can use a three-finger notch to test the same place—if it's a latch and not just a weak spot, a three-finger notch should test strong.

you continue along that line, you can find evidence of past lives when the Gatekeeper locked this issue into your soul's expression.

When I am clearing gating on myself, I love to tune in to the box to let it tell its stories, to give me insight into how this storyline played out for me. When I am working with clients, they often get a clear sense of what each latch relates to so I let them tell the stories.

To unlatch: Using your finger energy, sink down into the place where the latch is sitting. Wait until you feel your energy has connected with the latch and then gently swing or pop it open. It may help to picture one of those hasp-latches you see in hotel rooms, with a bar that swings across (see Figure 9.6).

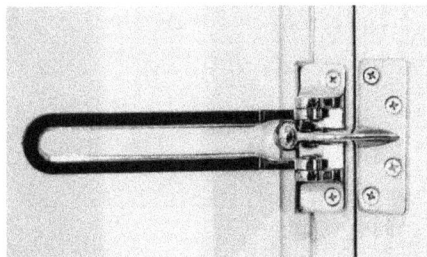

Figure 9.6. Hasp Latch

5. Dissolve the panel of the box.

Use the Divine Hook-Up (see page 37): Plug one index finger into Source and plug the other index finger or full palm into the side of the box. This will bring Radiance to the area to gently balance or dissolve this artifact of the Gatekeeper. Radiance does more than just dissolve the gating; it also brings healing energy to the self you were when the gating got set up!

6. Seal the Deal.

I generally reinforce the shift by tracing the five-element star (which reinforces control of energies) and the circle (which supports the flow of energies) over the area where the gate has been (see page 110).

7. Clear the next side of the box.

Proceed to the next side of the box, repeating steps 3 to 6.

Because you are working with your Gatekeeper, as you clear gating, check in periodically to see if you are experiencing any reactivity. If so, repeat the Porcupine Reset and trace hearts on your heart. The Gatekeeper sometimes gets triggered by too much change at once.

HEALING YOUR HARMONIC SELF

Sonya was much healed by reclaiming her Storymaker equipment and clearing distorted templates of learning with the Storyline Track and Balance work she did. And, in many ways, clearing the gating that had boxed her in essentially released her from bondage. But as we clear out old storylines, we need to make sure they aren't still in the archives somewhere.

Sonya spent most of her life living a set of stories that did not allow her to dream, fly, and experience her potential. She had codified these storylines into one more place within her energies: her harmonic self.

Your harmonic self is a kind of master blueprint that codifies who and how you are. I sometimes call it your "always self" because it holds steady the truths you have distilled about yourself, even in the face of contradictory information.

For example, if you have always had strong healthy teeth, but one day go to the dentist and discover a cavity, you think, *That's weird. I have great teeth. This is just an anomaly.* Another person who has a history of cavities goes to the dentist, discovers a new cavity, and thinks, *That figures. I've got terrible teeth.* These truths about yourself can change, but unless you have a lot of evidence to the contrary, the harmonic self holds an energetic blueprint for you that resists the ups and downs of day-to-day experience.

This is useful, in that your identity doesn't just blow with the wind or yield to other people's suggestions and perceptions of you. On the other hand, if your harmonic self has templates that don't serve you, it can hold those steady even in the face of new, improved information.

Sonya's harmonic self was riddled with templates that basically reinforced the message that the world is an unsafe place, that people can't be trusted, and that her membership in groups was never secure. It was also riddled with templates that instructed her Gatekeeper to keep the world at bay, no matter what her conscious mind thought it might like.

Although she transformed many of the templates she carried within her, she needed to bring transformation to her harmonic self as well. Most of us have not experienced the magnitude of trauma and betrayal that Sonya has, but we *have* had our own harsh lessons that left us with conclusions in our blueprints that we'd rather not leave in there guiding our life story.

And because the harmonic self blueprint reflects our efforts to create a self to meet the world we find ourselves in, in this era of awakening and breakdown, many of us carry scribbles that have crept into our harmonic selves that reflect a groupthink world we'd rather not be designed by. In other words, it might be worth your while to indulge in some refurbishment of your harmonic self!

Protocol: Refurbishing Your Harmonic Self

To access your harmonic self, you need to first open your cosmic gates. These are doorways between your *embodied self* and your more cosmic dimensions. When you are challenged in an existential way, or your Storymaker is not free to create fulfilling stories, your Gatekeeper can swing these cosmic gates shut and even lock them down. If that happens, your energies may not be able to hold their truth, keep their integrity, or withstand forces outside yourself. And your Storymaker may not have good access to your innate Radiance—the light of your consciousness. Your Storymaker *needs* that Radiance to write stories that are true to your deepest nature.

I think it's useful to have an image that helps you locate and interact with a particular energy. You will find your first cosmic gate at arm's length plus one foot in front of you. If you imagine a big egg more or less twelve inches larger than your body, that's about what the gate looks like to me.

On the other side of that first gate, you will find your *harmonic self*. At arm's length plus one foot beyond your harmonic self sits the second cosmic gate. On the other side of that second gate stands your *fully realized self*. See Figure 9.7 on the following page.

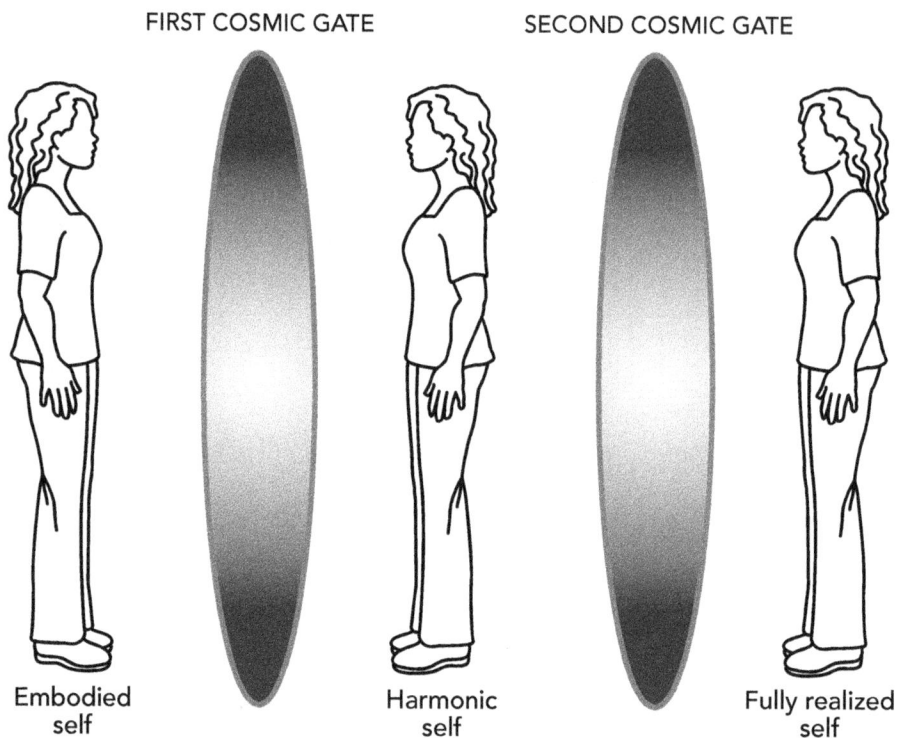

FIRST COSMIC GATE   SECOND COSMIC GATE

Embodied   Harmonic   Fully realized
self   self   self

Figure 9.7. Positions of the Cosmic Gates, the Embodied Self, the Harmonic Self, and the Fully Realized Self

To access your harmonic self, to explore your Field of Possibility, or just to make sure your Storymaker is getting inspired by your consciousness, it is important to unlock and open your cosmic gates. Here's how:

1. Reach out with your palm and *feel into the first gate*. You can use your intuition to determine whether the gate has been locked. If you are comfortable with energy testing (see Appendix A), you can do a polarity test: With your palm facing the gate, you should get a strong test. With the back of your hand facing the gate, you should get a weak test. Any other configuration means your gate has been locked.

2. *To unlock it*, reach out and use a gesture to grasp it top and bottom, like a large Frisbee. Inhale, and as you exhale, flip it, so the side that was facing you now faces away from you. This breaks any Gatekeeper seals

and calms your Gatekeeper whether or not the gate was locked down. So even if you don't know whether the gate was sealed, go ahead and flip the Frisbee.

3. Next, *unlatch it.* I always picture one of those hasp latches (see Figure 9.6 on page 249). But it's fine to see it as a doorknob or some other kind of latch. Again, using gesture, reach out, inhale, and unlatch the gate as you exhale (or turn the knob or flip the hasp).

4. Finally, inhale, and on the exhale, gently *push open the gate.* And greet your harmonic self, standing on the other side. You can figure-eight between your body (embodied self) and this master template to create rapport.

5. Invite your harmonic self to turn and help you open the second cosmic gate, at arm's length plus one foot beyond your harmonic self. Again, feel into whether the door is locked (or energy test). Reach out, grasp the gate top and bottom, inhale, and on the exhale, flip it like a Frisbee to *unlock it,* so the front is now the back.

6. Inhale, reach out to the latch, and on the exhale, *unlatch it.*

7. Finally, inhale, and on the exhale, *push open your second cosmic gate.* Take a moment to feel what arises for you with both gates open. And meet the being who is standing on the far side of the second gate: your fully realized self.

8. Figure-eight between your fully realized self and harmonic self, and then again, between your harmonic self and your embodied self. Feel the linkages between these dimensions of your being.

Now that your gates are open, you can interact with your harmonic self and your fully realized self and carry out some refurbishments. Here are some options:

Do a Suit Reboot on your embodied self. This is one of the first exercises my Councils ever taught me, to use when I needed to clear my tangled, glommed energies:

1. Imagine your body is a suit, like a big snowsuit.

2. Push back the hood, unzip your suit down the front, open the flaps.

3. Step forward, climbing out of the suit and leaving it standing behind you. Turn to face the suit you have left standing there.

4. Lean down to pick it up by the feet. Shake it out gently, like shaking wrinkles out of laundry.

5. Dip the suit in the "Well of Resolution" or a well filled with whatever quality you desire, such as love, grace, kindness, or forgiveness.

6. Set the suit back on its feet, smoothing up the legs and arms to make sure it is upright and open for you. Then turn, step back into your suit, pull up your hood, and zip up!

Note: Never abandon this exercise midstream. Without your suit, your Gatekeeper will definitely signal its displeasure with noticeable symptoms.

This pattern of opening your cosmic gates and then doing a Suit Reboot is a great way to open any session of exploring your Field of Possibility. (You do not need to close the cosmic gates afterward. Your Gatekeeper will close them as needed.)

Variation: After you have rebooted your embodied suit, step forward into the space with your harmonic self, and have both of you do a Suit Reboot together. Then invite your harmonic self to step forward with you into the realm of your fully realized self, and have all three Suit Reboot together. This gives your energies a multi-dimensional clearing and brings them into greater alignment. (This variation was offered by one of my students.*)

---

* Thanks to Stacy Newman for this innovation. It is always exciting to hear how people are taking this work and making it their own.

Further Energy Medicine to Do with Your Harmonic Self

With your cosmic gates newly opened, you can basically do any energy medicine you know on or for your harmonic self. Storymaker support is especially effective here. Do something that addresses framing, anchoring, weaving, sourcing, steering, and learning.

1. **Framing:** Figure-eight your harmonic self from top to bottom, then from side to side, and then do Expanding Hearts (see page 72) on your harmonic self.

2. **Anchoring:** Try holding some or all of the Storymaker anchors (see page 91) on your harmonic self. For some people, using gesture and miming this works very well, interacting with their harmonic self where it lives. But if that isn't comfortable for you, once your cosmic gates are open, you can also interact with your harmonic self eight inches above your body. To do this, hold your own anchor, for example, your physical left knee, with one hand, and with the other hand, hold your palm eight inches above the left knee, in harmonic resonance with the physical hold.

3. **Weaving:** Celtic-weave (see page 93) both your embodied self and your harmonic self. If your core weaves have been deeply disrupted, as Sonya's were, you may need to reinforce your harmonic self Body Weave (see page 158) or Safety Net (see page 189). To strengthen her Safety Net, Sonya held the Harmonizing Hook-Up (see page 195) on her harmonic self (right hand on the front of the left shoulder, left hand on the front of the left pelvis), and she asked her harmonic self to hold hands with her fully realized self to bring in Radiance. This significantly shifted her energies and allowed her to more easily clear templates relating to being safe in this world.

4. **Sourcing:** Refurbish your harmonic self's Umbilical Passage (see page 182) or Mingmen Passage (see page 186). For Sonya, the Umbilical Passage was key in starting to believe she could get her needs met.

5. **Steering:** Ask your harmonic self to turn around, so you can adjust its tailbone. Or reset its face and nose, as described on page 193.

6. Learning: Even though your harmonic self is a master template, you can also track and balance issues in its chakras. Rather than doing a full protocol there, I usually reach out with my right hand to cover each chakra in turn while saying, "Bring up all the templates related to *[my issue]*." Then I clear the templates using a Divine Hook-Up (see page 37). Because the harmonic self lives beyond your cosmic gate, you don't need to go down through layers to find their other dimensions. By meeting with them where they live, you are *in* their dimension!

When you have finished working with your harmonic self and fully realized self, Celtic-weave yourself and your harmonic self. Invite your fully realized self to Celtic-weave both you and your harmonic self.

PLAY IN YOUR FIELD OF POSSIBILITY

Once Sonya had finally been liberated from the Gatekeeper lockdown and templates that kept her from engagement with the world, she had the wonderful assignment of learning to play in her Field of Possibility—to explore her multi-dimensional self in that place where it was okay to try things on for size, to create and re-create, to let her imagination run wild and run deep.

And she took to it like a fish in water. After a lifetime of being shuttered and shattered by the collective reality she'd grown up in, she was able to take time and space to explore her own potential to create storyline and to find her inner and outer tribe. This is part of our work as souls-in-body, and although she got a late start, she soon discovered some of the counterpart selves and guides who gave her access to her larger wisdom.

There are many ways to play with the Field of Possibility, some more woo-woo than others. It is great to do any form of creative artwork, finding ways to explore the worlds that aren't reality but are real to you. And you can, of course, find endless possibilities while traveling and interacting energetically in the Country of the Mind, as I've shown you throughout this book.

One fun way to explore is to use the Storyline Track and Balance process to travel outward rather than inward. In other words, instead of taking the *down elevator* or finding passages taking you deeper within, take the *up elevator* (or escalator or any vehicle that appeals to you) to explore realms within your Field of Possibility. As I mentioned earlier, this field exists in many dimensions. I'm not going to try to pin down its architecture because that's not the path of wisdom. Travel in the Field of Possibility involves using launch places, not creating hierarchies.

But like what happens in a dream or in a creative story, you can explore your web of meaning here without the restrictions of needing to embody each story. Here's a guided visit to help you find your way to some launchpads.

Guided Visit: Explore Your Stories in the Field of Possibility

To get the most out of the guided visits in this book, you can either record the text for yourself, leaving silent spaces to allow yourself to explore as guided, or you can download an MP3 recording I've provided and use that. See page 13 for instructions on how to access the MP3s.

Note: I have incorporated the exercises Suit Reboot and Opening Your Cosmic Gates into this guided visit. Doing these will help you prepare to encounter the Field of Possibility.

Preliminary: Before you enter the Field of Possibility, it is helpful to balance your energies so that your body knows you are not asking it to enact what you experience there.

To calm any reactivity you might be feeling, pet yourself behind the ears (*good doggy, good kitty*). Breathe in through your nose on a count of three and out your mouth on a count of five to calm your body and mind.

Now, it's great to do a Suit Reboot to quickly reset all your energy systems. Imagine your body is a big, hooded snowsuit, like little kids wear to play in the snow. Reach up and push your hood back, unzip the front zipper, open the flaps, pull one arm out of the sleeve, then your other arm, and lift your legs out of each legging, one at a time. Turn to face your suit.

Reach down and grab both legs of your snowsuit, and dip it in a well of restorative, healing waters. You can imagine this well filled with any quality you'd like to imbue your suit with. Then gently shake it like shaking a sheet to get the wrinkles out, and stand it up in front of you, zipper facing you. Turn around, and step back into your suit, one leg at a time, one arm at a time. Pull the suit up, close the flaps, zip it up to your chin, and cover your head with the hood.

Now, we're going to open our cosmic gates. Reach out in front of you. At arm's length and one foot beyond is your first cosmic gate. Grasp it top and bottom to flip it, like a Frisbee, so the side that was facing you is now facing away. That will unlock the gate for you.

Now reach out again, take a deep breath in through your nose, and as you breathe out through your mouth, unlatch your cosmic gate, however you picture it opening. It might be a typical gate latch, a doorknob, or some other arrangement. On your next exhale, gently push the door open.

Greet your harmonic self, standing on the other side of the doorway. Figure-eight between you and your harmonic self. And ask them to turn and help you open the second cosmic gate, at arm's length plus one foot beyond where they are standing. Using your intention to reach out to the second gate, perhaps with the help of your harmonic self, grasp your second cosmic gate top and bottom, and flip the polarity, like a Frisbee, turning front to back.

Take a deep breath in through your nose, and as you exhale, reach out to unlatch this second gate. On your next exhale, open this gate . . . and greet your fully realized self, standing there. Figure-eight between your harmonic self and fully realized self, then figure-eight between both of those selves and your embodied self.

Now you are ready to play in the Field of Possibility. Feel free to invite your harmonic self and fully realized self to accompany you or to call upon your Councils or guides to come along if you wish. Or just go on your own, knowing you might meet others to play with.

The purpose of traveling into your Field of Possibility is to meet energies that are moving toward you, to create storylines and characters you'd love to have in your stories, to meet guides or inspiring souls, to work out plotlines in this place that supports you to experiment—or just to enjoy the journey.

Take a moment to consider how you'd like to travel. If you want to use the up elevator, imagine it in a place you are happy to launch from and return to. If you want to just discover passageways as you go, that is fine too. Or maybe you've got some kind of transport that comes to you as the way you want to move through this realm today.

If you prefer to use a chakra to travel through, just tune in to see which one you feel drawn to today. And, if you wish, you can ask for insight into a particular issue, or instead, just travel to see what shows up.

Now, step into your elevator or vehicle, or find your passageway, and move to the first floor, the first stop on your tour today.

Look around you, sense into where you find yourself. Who is there for you? What do you want or need as you bide in this place? What is your feeling about this visit? Are you here to learn something, to experience something, or to just have some fun? Ask the place what it offers you today or needs from you today. . . .

You can stay here as long as you'd like. If you feel like it, you can do some simple energy medicine, such as drawing the five-element star and circle. You can also do a Divine Hook-Up to bring Radiance to this space.

When you feel done with this stop on your journey, take a moment to jot down or voice record what you want to remember.

Then get in your elevator or vehicle and travel to the next place on your journey. Again, look around you and use all your senses to pick up what the story is here. You may find this place makes you feel different, has a different ambiance. What can you notice? Invite your Councils or fully realized self and harmonic self to explore this place with you.

Again, do a Divine Hook-Up and trace a five-element star and circle to help balance the energies here and support your embodied self.

When you feel done with this stop on your journey, take a moment to jot down or voice record what you want to remember.

Then get in your elevator or vehicle and travel to the next place. Explore, greet the consciousness you find there, and investigate the space. . . .

You may find at this point that you're done for today, in which case, you can get back in your elevator or vehicle and return to the ground floor. As you get familiar with the Field of Possibility, you will get a clearer sense of which floors are calling to you in each visit.

Once you are back at the ground floor or your starting place, thank all your guides and the souls you interacted with, and greet your body by placing both hands on your heart and breathing in through your nose on a count of three and out your mouth on a count of five.

* * *

Since the Field of Possibility is fluid, you don't need to worry about what each level means. In general terms, the first few levels relate to your own storylines and creation of self, the middle levels relate to your affinities and karmic connections with others, and the outer levels take you into the interface with other dimensions of reality.

Your Field of Possibility is not a place to map or catalog. It offers you access to the drawing board, where you can play, create, make meaning, and bring healing energy to your creation of self. It is a wonderful workspace to support you, not just in fixing what's wrong, but in creating a new world for yourself and others.

As you wind toward the end of this book, you might be wondering where this is going to land. Keep reading. We're almost there.

CHAPTER TEN

Creating a New World

"I'm glad you finished your book," said a friend of mine, "but I don't like to read books. I don't even want to learn how to heal myself. I want to come see you as a practitioner and have you put me right." Although I could empathize with that desire for someone to just fix her (I've been there!), I couldn't help but feel that impulse was part of the challenge for all of us. We want our world to be better, but we have also been conditioned into receptivity and passivity: to let other people set the agenda, do the work, and somehow, magically fix us.

If you are reading this chapter, chances are you're *not* one of the ones who doesn't read books or doesn't want to learn how to work with your own energies. I'm hoping the mix of stories and exercises will inspire you to experiment with your own Storymaker and explore your energies in a dynamic way.

Having said that, this may be new territory for you, with new terminology, even if you are familiar with energy medicine and energy healing. I have put a lot of thought into how to make this material accessible without dumbing it down! I'm hoping the combination of stories, written explanations, illustrations, and links to videos of the exercises and audio recordings of the guided visits will give you a fuller experience of your possibilities.

A more enthusiastic friend who actually read the book commented, "This is all great, but where do I start? Do you have some kind of a daily routine for the care and feeding of your Storymaker?"

My short answer to that was "no." The whole point of understanding that energy medicine is a form of communication is to recognize that the body does not necessarily love to have pat phrases thrown at it. It wants to be heard and responded to, not submitted to some kind of disciplined routine. (At least my body wants that.)

Be that as it may, I also know that sometimes it is good to have some way to get us past the passivity of doing nothing and not even wanting to engage in dialogue with the instruments of expression we inhabit. So the longer answer is "yes."

In this chapter, you'll find a short set of activities you can use if you want to find a time each day to invite your Storymaker to play and make it a more regular part of your routine. These exercises will help you anchor, frame, weave, source, steer, and learn from your subtle energies and will strengthen your Storymaker over time.

Protocol: A Daily Routine for Your Storymaker

Feel free to substitute other exercises from this book to help strengthen each of your Storymaker capacities. This set of practices can be done fairly quickly, like grabbing a quick energy snack. Or it can be done more slowly, like savoring a multicourse tasting menu to bring your Storymaker more fully into engagement. In most cases, it should take only five to ten minutes.

1. Anchoring

Start with a series of quick holds (for three deep breaths in through your nose and out through your mouth, or longer if desired):

➤ Hold both knees.

➤ Hold your **Mingmen area** behind your belly button on your back. If you can't reach, hold your belly button and send your intention back to the Mingmen.

➤ Hold the **bottoms (arches) of both feet.** Hold one at a time if you can't reach both at once. If you can't reach at all, place one foot on top of the other, so your arch can feel the contact of touch.

➤ Place both hands over your **heart chakra.**

➤ Hold the **sides of your face**, with your little fingers along your cheeks in line with the centers of each eye, and with your index fingers touching behind your ears and thumbs touching the sides of the neck. This grounds you and supports your vagus nerve.

➤ Hold your **thinking cap** with the heels of each hand above each ear, and your fingers extending upward to meet at the top of your head where the soft spot is on babies.

If you are comfortable doing the Storymaker Reset (see page 91), you can substitute it here.

2. Framing

Do a Smart Filter (see page 58) on the edge of your aura, weaving figure eights along the edge of your aura, toward and away from the body. As you figure-eight, weave into your smart filter one quality you would like to contribute to the shared culture today. Invite that quality in to help you frame your experiences and stories all day long.

3. Weaving

Commune with your Body Weave (see page 158) by holding each string of your *tennis racket* in turn and sending sound or color through it. "Tune Your Weave" is one powerful way to do this. See page 265 for instructions.

4. Sourcing

Use a Divine Hook-Up (see page 37) to fill your Mingmen Passage and Umbilical Passage with Radiance.

Plug your left index finger into the heart of the Divine, however you experience that, and use your right hand to juice up and activate your Mingmen Passage with Radiance. If you can't reach the Mingmen, just aim the energy in that direction while leaning on a pillow or some surface that allows you to feel that part of your back.

Then, keeping your left index finger plugged into the heart of the Divine, place your other hand or index finger on your belly button to juice up and activate your Umbilical Passage with Radiance.

5. Steering

Do a Harmonizing Hook-Up (see page 195) in silence for approximately three minutes. Place one hand flat over the front of your left pelvis and the other hand on the front of your left shoulder and arm seam. Imagine yourself wrapped in a rainbow hammock or wrap yourself in a multi-colored cloth.

Allow your energies to gather and come home until you feel your steering mechanisms (your Assemblage Point, your tailbone, your face, your heart and gut, and your third eye and gaze) reset. If you don't know what this feels like, just hold for three minutes or longer until you feel something settle into place within you.

6. Learning

Do the exercise Heaven and Earth Tuning (or Do-Re-Mi Chakras, page 265). In general, similar to how you reinforced your Body Weave, you are going to hold each of the seven chakras in turn, starting with your root chakra, while singing a scale upward, one note per chakra. Since the scale has eight notes, you'll sing the last note while reaching toward the sky. Then you'll reverse the process: starting your top note while holding your crown chakra, and singing down the scale, with one note per chakra, until you sing the last note while reaching downward toward the earth.

7. Reinforcing Your Storymaker's Evolution

End your energy routine by Celtic-weaving (see page 93) your body and field.

Exercise: Tune Your Weave

1. Start on one note for the first strand, and then sing up the scale for each subsequent strand. On the eighth note, reach out your arms to hug the world.

2. Then, reverse direction, and while holding strings 7-6-5-4-3-2-1, in turn, sing the scale back downward. On the final note, hug yourself.

3. Figure-eight across your body at the hips, waist, rib cage, and shoulder seams (where the arms connect to the body) to strengthen your horizontal strings.

Because each note of the musical scale corresponds to an energy system in the body, singing the scale as you reinforce your Body Weave aligns your energy systems with one another and anchors them into your foundation.

If singing is hard for you, you can use a recorded scale. Or try using colors of the rainbow to infuse each string with color, in this sequence: purple—indigo—blue—green—yellow—orange—red. As with sound, hug the world at the top of the rainbow, and hug yourself at the bottom.

• • •

Exercise: Heaven and Earth Tuning

This exercise integrates your chakra energies with your energy systems and balances them between heaven and earth. This helps you codify your learning and experience your stories, past and present, in a more balanced way.

Here are step-by-step instructions:

1. Start by placing your hand flat over your root chakra at the base of your torso. Sing the first note of a scale while you hold your root chakra. (You will be singing the whole scale, so start at a note that is low enough.)

2. Then hold your second (sacral) chakra, and sing the next note upward on your scale.

3. Move your hand to your third (solar plexus) chakra, and sing the next note upward on your scale.

4. Continue, moving up to your fourth (heart), fifth (throat), sixth (third eye), and seventh (crown) chakras, holding each and singing the next note upward on the scale.

5. Stretch your hand upward toward the heavens, and sing the top, eighth note of the scale.

6. Then to start singing the scale back down, place your hand back on your seventh chakra and sing that same top note of your scale while holding your crown.

7. Proceed downward, singing each note of the scale downward while holding your sixth, fifth, fourth, third, second, and first chakras in turn. Sing the *final* starting note of your scale while reaching downward toward the earth.

* * *

CODA

It was a gorgeous spring day in Southern California, the kind where the blue of the sky is almost liquid. This was around 2012, and I was in a museum to see a visiting exhibition of terracotta figures from five centuries in China. I remember walking along, communing with a few figures, then pausing to stare out the window at the unusually clear sky. I was wired for sound, listening to the explanations of what I was seeing. Then suddenly, I was energetically whacked. I could barely stand up, felt dizzy and disoriented, completely discombobulated.

I stumbled my way to a bench in the corner to assess my energies. They had come completely unglued—in a pattern I call a "cosmic whack"—so I set about quietly reinstating my balance, pulling everything back into communication again. Fortunately, the museum was nearly empty that day. When I looked up, a Chinese gentleman was standing in front of me—a spirit—sporting a long, thin beard, wearing a floor-length brown robe, like one of the clay figures come to life.

For a few years, in the early days of my practice, I had worked with a spirit I called the Old Chinese Gentleman, who would show up when I was in sessions with clients to suggest ways to help them. I've spoken about him earlier in this book. He taught me a technique I jokingly called "ghost acupuncture."

This spirit looked old, but younger and rounder than my Old Chinese Gentleman. He said, "My grandfather asked me to contact you." As he spoke, I realized he was the Old Chinese Gentleman's grandson. "He would like to know if you will work with him again. He has some techniques and material he would like to pass on."

"Was that you who created the disruption in my energies?" I asked.

"Yes, my apologies," he replied. "I wanted to get your attention."

"Why didn't he come himself?" I asked.

"He is getting ready to pass on to another dimension, from which he will not be able to communicate directly. Before he leaves, he would like to be in contact with you."

"Yes," I said, "of course. I would be delighted to see him again."

The spirit bowed and disappeared. I managed to re-establish my balance and continued on my visit, bemused at the formality of this request from a spirit who had regularly dropped in unannounced back in the day.

A few nights later, the Old Chinese Gentleman appeared as a shadowy presence, with his grandson along as a messenger. He offered me a technique the grandson referred to as "The Four Stabilizing Colors." As with his other work, clients responded well to the technique, and I found it helped seal in other energy work and stabilize the body. (See Appendix B for an explanation of this exercise.)

And then, a month later, on the eve of a trip I was planning to take to Scandinavia, they again appeared at night as I was reading in bed. This time, the Old Chinese Gentleman was even more shadowy. And the grandson said, "My grandfather has a body of work he wants to pass on, if you will accept it." (As if I'd refuse an offer like that.)

I asked him if he could tell me anything about the work.

He replied, "My grandfather was a renowned healer and scholar at a time in China just prior to when the five elements became more developed. He bridged many worlds and philosophies and has worked with healers from many cultures to refine his understandings. He would like to pass this on to you, not as a historical document, but to be translated into contemporary terms and context."

I didn't want to be rude, but I was thinking, *Why me? Couldn't he have found a Chinese medicine scholar who would know what to do with this stuff?*

The grandson must have been able to read my thoughts. Well, since I was conversing with him in my imagination, I guess thoughts and statements were pretty much the same thing! He said, "You have ties to his lineage and are in a position to do this work. It may take several years to unfold."

I tend to leap first and ask questions about what it will entail later, so I said, "Sure, I'd be honored to accept this task."

They both bowed.

Then the grandson handed me a miniature lacquered jewel case, with a curved top and elaborate decorations (an energetic jewel case, of course) and said, "He has coded the teachings onto seven grains of rice. When you are on your voyage, choose a good moment, and take one grain of rice under your tongue. Let it dissolve fully. Then wait, perhaps a full twenty-four hours, before you take the next one. They must all be assimilated while you are on your journey."

Hmmm, I wondered, *why is that?* Sometimes these spirit conversations don't lend themselves to closer questioning on details.

I repeated the instructions. They both bowed again and then faded away.

Two weeks later, riding on a bus in Finland, approaching the Arctic Circle, I felt a kind of *ping* inside me: It was time to eat the first grain of rice. I felt ridiculous and frankly a titch nervous, but I quietly opened the jewel case, chose one of the grains, and put it under my tongue.

And felt . . . strange sensations, like a movie playing two rooms over, where you can't hear or see it, but you know a story is being told. It was not uncomfortable, but it was odd to feel the energies assimilating into me. I could tell it was being stored in my being but not yet unpacked.

I'm not one of those people who use the term "download" to refer to channeled material. I feel it is a dismissive way to talk about what I see as a learning process and a more dynamic dialogue with teachers. Just getting information, like downloading a file from the internet, does not confer knowledge or wisdom. Channeling, in my experience, activates changes within the person receiving the guidance or contact; it is interactive.

But this felt closer to a download of a file—one I knew was zipped and would unpack and install later. Unlike downloading a file, however, I did get a shadowy sense of what this was. Not information, not culturally linked material, but a sense of frameworks and processes and essences. I can't explain why, but it felt shamanic and animistic in nature, yet mathematical and organized, ancient and modern—or maybe outside of time.

I sat on the bus, pretending to watch the scenery, thinking, *Oh crap, what have I taken on here?* I jokingly started thinking of it as pregnant rice. And each day, as we transferred from the bus to a boat and made our way down the coast from Finland to Norway, past breathtaking vistas, I would choose what felt like the right moment to privately, ceremonially, dissolve another grain of pregnant rice under my tongue.

And that was it. When I finished the last grain, the lacquer case just melted away.

Over the next six months, I had frequent bouts of Z flu. My Councils explained that my system was being prepared and rewired to handle the new energies coded into the rice, so I tried not to worry about what was growing in me, and went about my business.

And since that time, I periodically find myself knowing something that I didn't learn directly. Something that has a certain character and feel to it. And I know it is from the Old Chinese Gentleman's gift. The charge was always to translate the knowledge into contemporary terms—not to reconstruct an ancient healing practice. In fact, I have gathered that pieces of this work derived from many different cultures and times, from lifetimes in which the spirit I knew as the Old Chinese Gentleman was learning his craft, evolving his frameworks, and shaping his style.

And what is this style? Usually simple, elegant, sometimes deceptively low-key. A framework for understanding. A technique that does not require much technical know-how. And I'm not even convinced that there *is* material or subject matter. It may, in fact, be a way of seeing and understanding life, energy, and the world that he was trying to pass on.

This book was born from the perspectives that were coded into those grains of rice. It is not a systematic inventory or rendition; rather, it's an attempt to bring you, the reader, into the wisdom and understanding the Old Chinese Gentleman wished to pass on to those who choose to receive it. May the words in this book become your pregnant rice, awakening you to your own history and wisdom, to your own tribes and kin within the World Wise Web. May you dance and play with your energies and find ways to individually and jointly create a new world.

Three Simple
Energy Self-Tests

The best way to test energies is to use your intuition and take soundings. But sometimes it is good to have feedback from the body in more physical terms. This is especially helpful when you want to determine whether an energy is strong (flowing adequately) or weak (obstructed or not flowing adequately). These three self-test options are easy to learn. They are meant to give you feedback and to amplify what energies are communicating, not to act as right-answer guides.

Although for each test in this appendix there is a clear "strong" and "weak" indication, if you pay attention, the energy test can show you some nuance: "Strong, but barely holding" feels different from "strong and resilient" and from "unbelievably strong—must be Gatekeeper interfering with the test."

The best way to develop confidence with your energy testing, which is a bit of an art form, is to practice with statements you think you know to be true or false, such as "My name is Ellen" or "Today is Tuesday " or "I am standing by a window."

Before you energy test, make sure you are hydrated, centered, and have a clear mind. To get feedback on the energies in a particular area, "energy localize" by touching that area.

THE BOTTLE TEST

1. Fill a large bottle or pitcher with water until it weighs enough that it is easy to pick up if you say something true, and harder to pick up if you say something clearly untrue. To check this (and to do the energy test), place the bottle on a table or shelf where you basically have to reach out at arm's length to grasp the neck or handle. (The goal is to get your arm more or less parallel to the floor as a starting place.)

2. Then make your statement (e.g., "My name is Ellen"), and immediately try to lift the bottle. It should be easy to lift with a true statement. Now, try it with a false statement (e.g., "My name is Mergatroyd.") It should be more difficult to lift with a false statement.

3. You can then use this bottle lift as an energy test while touching (energy localizing) the thing you want to test. You can also use it while keeping situations in mind when you want the body's input about whether or not the energies are flowing well within those situations. The more abstract the query, though, the less likely your body will be able to respond accurately. That's why energy localizing is a safer bet.

4. For energy testing where the storyline lives, you would touch each chakra in turn and say, "Show me a weak test if there are templates for [name your issue] here." To determine which chakra is juiciest, you can then touch each chakra where the storyline lives to say, "Show me a weak test if this is the priority place to track [name your issue]."

5. The reason you are asking to be shown a weak test is to specify that you are looking for templates and not an overall weather report on the flow of energies in the chakra.

6. For energy testing whether one of your body's polarities is reversed (our bodies are very electrical and have plus/minus polarities throughout), energy localize with your palm facing (near or touching) the area while you lift your bottle to test. If the polarity is correct, you should get a *strong* test. If you flip your hand, so the back is facing the same area, you should get a *weak* test. Any other result indicates a disturbed polarity. You can energy localize for polarities using any energy test.

FINGER EXTENSION TEST

I tend to use the finger extension test most frequently because it can be done one-handed and subtly.

Extend your index finger so it is straight. Then, using your middle finger on the same hand, place the middle fingertip on the nail of the index finger, or if it is more comfortable, farther back toward the knuckle. Press downward on the index finger with your middle finger.

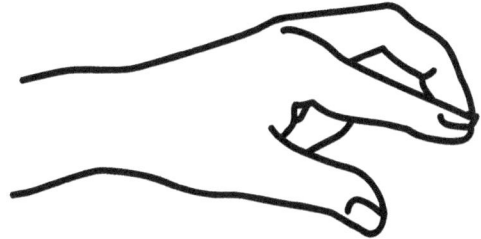

Figure A.1. Finger Extension Test

If it holds its strength, that is a strong test, and if it releases its hold, that is a weak test, showing disrupted flow. This energy self-test can also be used for testing your storyline and polarities.

FINGER CIRCLE TEST

Make a circle with your thumb and index finger or thumb and middle finger. Create an interlocking circle with the thumb and index or middle finger of the other hand. Use the thumb and index finger of your other hand to try to pull the two circles apart while saying your statement: "Show me a weak test if this is the priority place to track [name your issue]."

If the circles stay linked, that is a strong response. If the circles come apart, that is a weak test showing disrupted flow, or in this case, a priority place to track your issue.

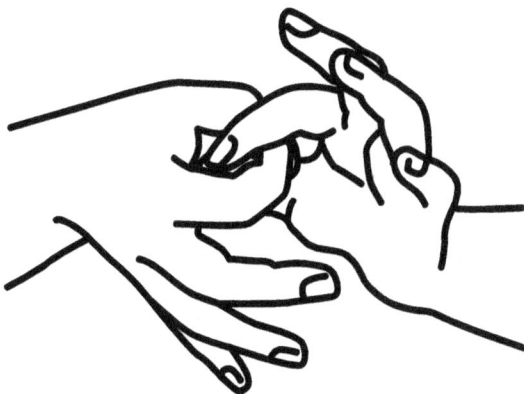

Figure A.2. Finger Circle Test

Since this test requires two hands, you can just touch each chakra or your target area with the edge of one of your hands while you do the test. Or you can touch the place and then test quickly after that. This test can also be used to check polarities. After energy localizing with your palm (either hand) immediately do this test. If you don't test right away, however, you won't get an accurate test.

Exercise: The Four Stabilizing Colors

This was the exercise given to me by the Old Chinese Gentleman, mentioned in chapter 10. I use it after any major healing session to stabilize my client's energies. I also use it on myself as a stand-alone activity when I'm feeling wobbly or off-balance. This pattern works to stabilize your whole body, or you can do it in miniature around the four corners of an organ to stabilize its function.

1. Using the four corners of the torso (front of right hip, front of right shoulder, front of left shoulder, and front of left hip,), place either hand flat on each position, starting with the front of the right hip and the color yellow. Imagine your body and entire field filling with *yellow* light.

2. When you feel full, move your hand to the second position, front of right shoulder, and imagine your body and aura filling with *red* light.

3. When that is full, move to position three, front of left shoulder, place your hand flat, and imagine your body and aura filling with *black* light, the dark of the night sky.

4. When that is full, move to position four, front of left hip, place your hand flat, and imagine your body and aura filling with *blue* light.

Try it to see what this feels like energetically. To bring further integration to the new stabilized state, if you wish, Celtic-weave your torso.

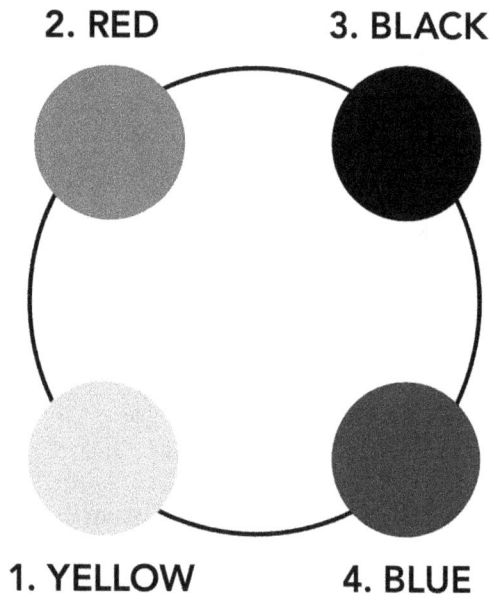

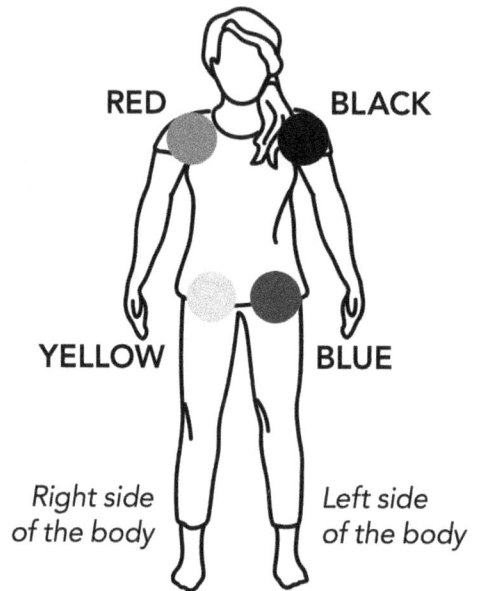

Figure B.1. The Four Stabilizing Colors

Daily Routine Protocol Sheet

Protocol: A Daily Routine for Your Storymaker

1. Anchoring

Quick holds (for three deep breaths): both knees, Mingmen area, bottoms of both feet, heart chakra, sides of your face, thinking cap.

2. Framing

Do a Smart Filter on the edge of your aura. Weave into your smart filter one quality you would like to contribute to the shared culture today.

3. Weaving

Holding each string of your Body Weave in turn, sing a scale up, one note per string, starting on left. On the eighth note upward, *hug the world*. Then starting with string seven, sing the scale back down, on the eighth note, *hug yourself.*

Alternative: Use colors in this order: purple—indigo—blue—green—yellow—orange—red.

Figure-eight across your body at the hips, waist, rib cage, and shoulder seams.

4. Sourcing

Use a Divine Hook-Up to infuse your Mingmen Passage and Umbilical Passage with Radiance.

5. Steering

Do a Harmonizing Hook-Up in silence for one to three minutes. Place one hand flat on your left shoulder and one hand flat on your left pelvis. Imagine yourself wrapped in a rainbow cloth.

Allow your energies to gather and come home until you feel your steering mechanisms (Assemblage Point, tailbone, face, heart and gut, third eye, and gaze) reset.

6. Learning

Do Heaven and Earth Tuning: Hold each chakra in turn, starting with your root chakra, while singing a scale upward, one note per chakra. Sing the last note while reaching toward the sky. Then starting your top note while holding your crown chakra, sing down the scale. Sing the last note while reaching downward toward the earth.

7. Reinforcing Your Storymaker's Evolution

Do a Celtic Weave to bring your energies into coherence.

List of Exercises, Protocols, and Guided Visits

Guided Visits

* Exercise reprised from earlier books with new applications.

Acknowledgments

Each of us relates in our own way to our inner life and our outer circumstances. I have been blessed in this life to find many teachers I call "inner teachers" and a good number of like-minded others with whom I could form my World Wise Web and my family of choice. Although I am more of an extrovert than introvert, when things get tough, my instinct is to go inward for reassurance, guidance, inspiration, and a sense of connection. That has served me well. So, I want to thank my Councils and my World Wise Web, including the Tibetans, for their support and fifty-plus years of guidance in exploring the *Country of the Mind.* You have opened my Michigan-trained brain to possibilities I needed to imagine, for the good of my soul and for the good of the planet.

In this long process, my wife, Judith, has been a constant and an anchor. I am so grateful for the adventures, the travel, and the daily thrum of living we have shared. I have known this beautiful soul through many lifetimes and feel so grateful we got to build a family and life together in this one.

I believe we each have many soulmates—those people whose Wiser Self shares the same Councils, the same cosmic purpose. It has been a delight to meet up with several in this life. In particular, Donna Eden has been such a loving and supportive fellow traveler. I am grateful for her mentoring, her friendship, her light, and her laughter. The energy medicine in this book is both Eden-inspired and "Eden-adjacent"—and should speak on many levels to anyone who follows Donna's brilliant, pioneering form of energy medicine.

Although they are thanked in footnotes, Stephanie Eldringhoff, Paulette Taschereau, Sandy Wand, Sara Allen, Sarah J. Buck, DeeAnn Weir Morency, and Stacy Newman deserve more thanks here. They each contributed insights and innovations (sometimes unknowingly) to this work.

When I was ready to find a home for this book, three fellow authors, Dr. Christine Horner, Dr. Anne Deatly, and our daughter, Dr. Gwen J. Bass, suggested I think outside the box and consider publishing alternatives. Within two days, I was given recommendations for two excellent possibilities. The first, a hybrid press dedicated to spiritual work, was run by a woman who had the same name as my paternal grandmother: Rosenau. The second possibility, an experienced team called The Book Couple, had the same name as my maternal grandmother: Rosenberg. The Universe has certainly learned how to get my attention!

After much deliberation (and advice from a friend, who asked, "Which was your favorite grandmother?"), I chose the Book Couple. What a GREAT choice! Carol Killman Rosenberg did an excellent job editing and shaping, and Gary Rosenberg designed the beautiful work you see in front of you. Larissa Henoch provided the wonderful illustrations. And the Book Couple guided me through the many details of book creation, providing excellent resources, such as Kim Weiss, for guidance on getting the book into the world, proofreader Lori Lewis, and indexer Kitty Chibnik. My grandmas (both of them) would have liked this personalized approach to book publishing—I certainly did. Thanks also to my team at Horse Mountain Press (my own imprint) for taking care of getting this book into people's hands.

I want to thank my book launch team for reading the galleys and preparing to write reviews, and thanks to all the generous souls who offered endorsements. Gratitude to print-on-demand outlets, which make book publishing a more accessible activity and save some trees in the process.

Gratitude to Richard Lalli, who always keeps me laughing; my L-group; my Victoria Community; the Chet-gals; Unity friends; my sister Marty and niece Bonnie; Kathy Lewis and Judith Evans for feedback on my first draft; and our son, Dan Evans, who manages my website, including the access to exercises and guided visits. Thanks to Barbara Allen, DC, who gave me my first work as a medical intuitive, and to Irene Young, photographer, for the back cover photo and my website design; thanks to Carol Ehrlich for website graphic design.

Special shoutout to the many teachers and practitioners of Eden Energy Medicine who supported my growing work, and who are themselves out there teaching, writing, and re-imagining the work of healing: Deborah Hurt, Melanie Smith, Lauren Walker, Madison King, Susan Stone, Anne Deatly, Sara Allen, Marjorie Fein, Janel Volk Hubbard, Amy MacDowell, Janie Chandler, Shura Gat, Ingrid de Geus, and Kathy Chambers, to name just a few. Special thanks to Tracy Stoves, who created and moderates my Facebook group: Energy Medicine with Ellen Meredith. Come check out how others are using and transforming the work I've birthed.

And gratitude to the more than 10,000 clients I was blessed to work with, and particularly to the souls who allowed their stories to be used (names and identifying details changed) in this book.

If I forgot to mention you, please know, you are still important—it takes many strands and weavers to create the Web of Connections.

Index

About the Author

Ellen Meredith, DA, is a conscious channel, medical intuitive, energy medicine practitioner, teacher, and author. She has been in practice since 1984, helping over 10,000 clients and students across the globe tune in to and communicate with their own energies, hear their inner guidance, and heal.

Ellen is renowned for her down-to-earth, yet out-of-the box thinking. Originally trained as a healer by her inner teachers (Councils), Ellen later became an Eden Energy Medicine Advanced Practitioner (EEMAP) and is an emeritus member of Donna Eden's faculty. She also serves on the faculty of Shift Network.

Ellen brings humanity, humor, and insight in many forms to the world of energy healing. Her approach to self-healing with energy medicine offers students ways to understand and get to the heart of their health and life challenges, and work compassionately with their body, mind, and spirit. She builds on everyday experiences and commonsense frameworks, believing that life reveals more of its meaning if you treat it as an evolving story and see yourself as a unique character helping to co-create it.

Your Body Lives Your Story: Energy Medicine to Heal Your Storymaker (Horse Mountain Press, 2025) is Ellen's fourth book on spiritual development and energy medicine. It follows *Your Body Will Show You the Way: Energy Medicine for Personal and Global Change,* Foreword by Lauren Walker (New World Library, 2022), *The Language Your Body Speaks: Self-Healing with Energy Medicine,* Foreword by Donna Eden (New World Library, 2020), and *Listening In: Dialogues with the Wiser Self* (Horse Mountain Press, 1993).

Although each book stands on its own, read together (in chronological order), they offer an original and extensive curriculum in self-healing and energy medicine for those who want to deepen their understanding of this emerging way to work with our mind-body-spirit construction of self.

Ellen has also created and filmed several intermediate and advanced energy medicine courses available for download or on DVD: *Energy Fluency, Gatekeeper, Storyline Track and Balance, Energy Chiro, Energy Wisdom, Healing Spaces, Intuition and Practitioner's Mind,* and *In Search of Radiance: Learning to Stand with your Wiser Self.*

Ellen lives in the Bay Area of Northern California with her wife and two cats. Visit her at www.ellenmeredith.com, and follow her on YouTube: @ellenmeredith.

For access to videos and MP3s, visit:
www.EllenMeredith.com/storyline (for password, see page 13)

(for password, see page 13)

www.ingramcontent.com/pod-product-compliance
Lightning Source LLC
Chambersburg PA
CBHW080245030426
42334CB00023BA/2701